Boys Talk

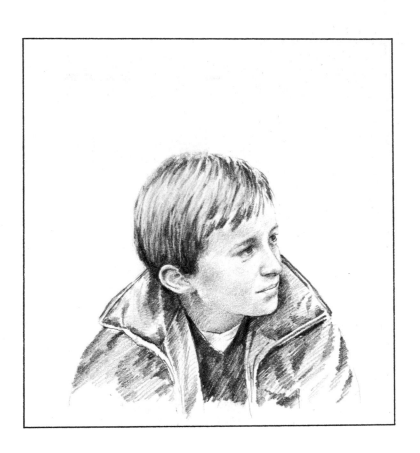

Boys Talk

Lucienne Pickering

GEOFFREY CHAPMAN
LONDON

Uniform with this book

*Girls Talk
Parents Listen*

A Geoffrey Chapman book published by
Cassell Ltd.
1 Vincent Square, London SW1P 2PN

First published 1981
Reprinted 1983, 1984
Reprinted with corrections 1986
British Library Cataloguing in Publication Data
Pickering, Lucienne
Boys talk.
1. Sex instruction
I. Title
616'.6007   HQ56

ISBN 0 225 66309 0

Diagrams by Illustra Design
Other illustrations by Alan Nivern
The illustrations on page 58 and page 59, top, are
based on illustrations in Gordon Bourne,
Pregnancy (Cassell, 1984) and used by per-
mission.
Printed and bound in Hungary at Kossuth Press
Contractors: I.P.V. Vue Touristique Publishing House Budapest

*For you
for today
and tomorrow*

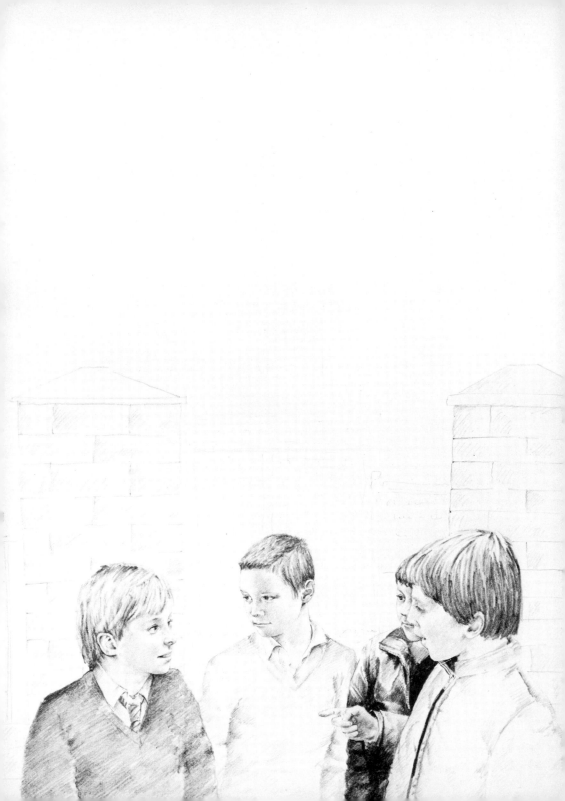

1

It was springtime. The four boys came out of school together. They always did: Andy, Nick, Pete and Tony had been friends since they began in primary school.

"Coming out tonight?" asked Andy.

"Where to?"

"Just out. Someone's put a rope on that old oak in the park. You can swing over the stream now."

"Magic. See you down there."

The friends broke up and went different ways. There was no need for more talk or firm arrangements. It was always like this – easygoing, friendly – explanations were never necessary. If you could come out, you did; if you couldn't, no one minded. After all, everyone had parents, so they all knew the kind of obstacles that were put in the way of their freedom.

Pete's dad would decide to have an enquiry into homework occasionally and deliver one of his serious talks on growing-up and not always 'messing around doing nothing with the boys'. "Find something useful," he would say, "give a hand around the house".

When he went in, his mother invariably said, "You're late, talking again I suppose, I don't know what you'll do when you really have to work." He was never quite sure if that was a question or an argument. Best to keep out of arguments and the best way to do that is to keep out of the house.

*   *   *

Pete is just a typical boy growing up. You and your friends are all about the same age as Pete and his friends. Your happiest times are when you are together. You enjoy freedom and getting away from authority, which at the moment probably means school and parents.

It was not always like this. There was a time when you were little and you felt safest close to your parents. Home was where you could be yourself; it was safe to be naughty, you knew all the rules. It was also safe because you knew you were loved. Your parents gave you lots of time and love. They taught you many things about talking, about playing, about looking after yourself.

Going visiting was another kind of adventure. You had to learn to play with other children. Some you liked and looked forward to seeing, others you had fights with: you did not like them and they did not like you. The world was not like home, full of friendly people.

However, because your parents still went on loving you, you learnt that it didn't matter if some boys didn't like you – that was their problem. You knew you were likeable because your parents told you so by the way they loved and cared for you.

This was a very important lesson for you to learn from your parents. It will help you through the next few years.

The 'next few years' are contained in words like 'teenagers' and 'adolescence' and stranger words like 'puberty'. You have probably heard them all at different times. They mean, very simply, the 'inbetween years': the time when you are no longer a young boy and not yet a man. They are important years because many changes will take place in you, in your body and in your mind.

You will have many questions you will want answered about you and your feelings, about girls and how they change and become women, about love and this word sex that all the boys seem to joke about.

It is possible that you have already seen films about these subjects at school, or maybe had talks from a teacher or a nurse or a marriage counsellor. Over the years, many of the questions may have been answered in part by your parents. You may talk to your friends about these matters and so share all the little bits of information gathered from older brothers and sisters, or by listening to adults talking.

Eventually it is necessary for you to put it all together and sort it into some kind of order that makes sense for your own life.

That is what this book is for. It does not expect to surprise you with all sorts of new facts, but it is going to attempt to state clearly and progressively how a boy develops and becomes a young man. When you first read it, just take in what you need to know and see if you can decide whereabouts you are, and what stage in your growth you have reached.

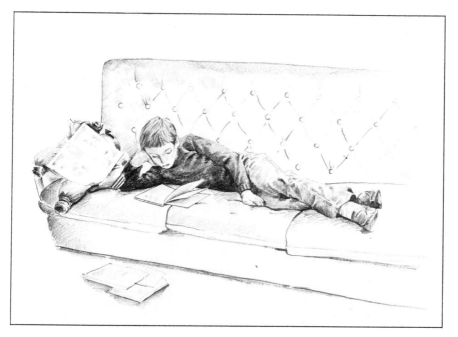

Afterwards keep it on your bookshelf in your bedroom and use it whenever you need to check some information. Maybe friends will ask you something about themselves, or maybe they will say things which you doubt or disagree with or want to find out if they are true. Everything in this book is reliable information and you can use it with confidence.

If your parents bought it for you, this is like giving you permission to talk about these matters to them. They are saying 'here is a book which says everything we would like to say to you. It has the right words and explanations, and we hope it will help you to understand some very important facts about your life.'

All about your body

When you learn human biology in school you will hear words used like 'organs' of the body and 'reproductive' systems. Many of the names used will be strange foreign words, mostly Latin or Greek. We don't have English words to substitute for these and so doctors continue to use the foreign names.

Boys have plenty of nicknames for parts of the body and no doubt you use these talking to your friends. However, here we will use the proper names so that if you ever needed to ask a doctor about yourself, you would have the right words and you would know what he or she was talking about.

There are also some diagrams in the book which will all be labelled with the correct names. Diagrams are used to show how things work. They are better than photos because a diagram can show inside something. Whenever you buy a machine of any kind or a car or model, you will be given a labelled diagram, so that you can understand how it works and look after it properly.

If you understand about your body you can care for it and if anything seems to be at fault you can explain to the doctor what and where the trouble is.

It is an important step towards growing up, to understand about yourself. Knowledge gives you independence, for as long as you have to ask other people you are dependent upon them. So it is a good thing to know and understand about yourself: it makes you confident and removes your fears and worries.

What you learn in this book is only a very simple explanation of those parts of you which are involved in your development from boy to man. You will learn in much greater detail at school about the functions of each part of your body.

For instance, the heart and veins and arteries are organs to do with blood circulating in you.

The stomach and liver and bowel are organs to do with food and digestion.

The lungs and windpipe are organs to do with breathing.

It is not necessary to know how they work now, but it is a simple fact that they work exactly the same and look exactly the same in men and in women.

The sex organs, however, are different in a man and a woman. They work differently and they look different.

The female sex organs are all to do with girls growing into women and the male sex organs are to do with boys becoming men.

Both male and female sex organs are part of the 'reproductive system'. They are the parts of your body concerned with reproducing life. There is no other way in which new life can be created than the way designed and built into your nature. This places a great responsibility on men and women. Their responsibility is firstly in bringing about the birth of new life and in caring for and looking after the young child; secondly, it is to pass this knowledge and wisdom to the next generation so that they in turn will know the importance and dignity of being parents.

That is another reason why your parents bought this book for you, and want you to read and think about these matters seriously.

Look first at this familiar sketch of a man. You have certainly seen your father undressed and probably boys of your own age, at the

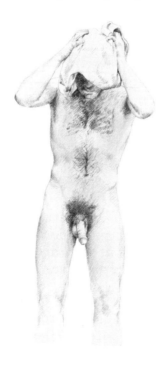

swimming baths or in the showers. You may have a younger brother with whom you share a room.

They all have, clearly visible, the male sex *organs*. There is a long fleshy tube properly called the 'penis'. This hangs down between the legs in front of the scrotum. Inside the scrotum are the testicles.

The next picture is a diagram of these parts, showing how these organs would look if you could see inside a man. Everything is labelled and you will notice how strange and foreign many of the words seem. Take some time to read and pronounce the words.

Now find each of these words on the following pages and read carefully what is their special work in your body.

Male sex organs
(side view)

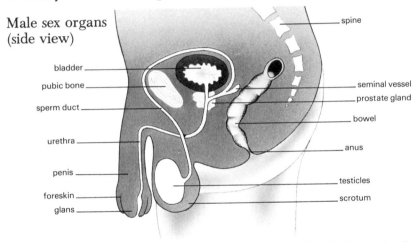

The bladder is like a reservoir for the waste fluid from the body. When you pass water it empties itself through the urethra, a tube from the bladder passing through the middle of the penis.

The bowel deals with the solid waste matter from the body. It expels this unwanted material through the anus. That is the back passage between the buttocks. It has nothing to do with the sex organs or reproduction – it is part of the digestive system in your body.

The penis is a soft fleshy organ that usually hangs down between the legs and below the abdomen. It is used from birth for passing out the waste liquids in the body, by means of the urethra.

The penis has a second very important job, such an important one that it only becomes able to perform this work when you become a man. It is the passage by which new 'life-cells' are passed.

The soft thick fleshy part of the penis which surrounds the urethra is made up of tissue which contains thousands of tiny spaces. When blood flows through and fills these spaces, the penis becomes fuller and firmer and longer. It becomes 'erect'. Then it no longer hangs limply between the legs, but firm and upright. This only happens at certain times which are explained farther on in this book.

The glans is the smooth round tip of the penis. It is covered by a 'foreskin'.

When you wash these parts of your body you should pull back the foreskin to expose the glans, which should be washed and kept clean to avoid becoming itchy and sore.

Sometimes, in a baby, the foreskin is too tightly joined over the glans and will not pull back. Mothers often discover this when they are bathing their little boys. Then the doctor must be told because he can put it right. He does a little operation which cuts away the skin round the glans – this operation is called circumcision.

Among the Jews and Arabs all boys are circumcised. It is a part of the religious custom. Some people choose to have this done because they think it more hygienic. Whether you are circumcised or not makes no difference to the way the penis works.

The scrotum is a skin bag which hangs behind the penis and is well protected by the legs. It has two sections divided by a thin membrane or tissue. In each section is a gland called a testicle.

You can feel these testicles with your hand, they are like two small marbles: boys often just call them 'balls' but their proper name is 'testicles'.

The seminal vessel and the prostate gland are small glands with a special job to do in the creating of life – which, you will recall, is what the sex organs are all about. Only the sex organs are concerned in reproducing life and they are the essential part of man. That is they give to you the special function which makes you a man, and manly, and enables you to be a father.

13

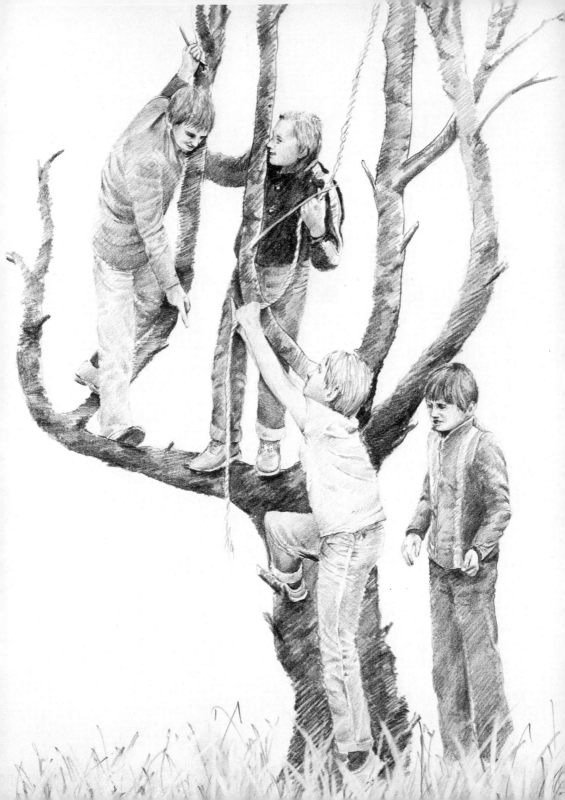

2

Nick made several attempts to pull himself up the rope onto the broad branch of the tree. The others fell about laughing at him.

"You should eat up your spinach, Nick."

"When are you going to start growing?"

"Muscles like sparrows' knee-caps, my Dad says!"

Nick took the banter in good humour, but wished he was as tall and strong as his friends. When they eventually got seated in the tree they talked about this.

"My Dad's so strong he moves furniture about like matchboxes. I wouldn't like to get on the wrong end of one of his punches."

"Is that how he manages to tame you?!"

"Well, it's a consideration: you don't argue with a sledge-hammer."

"My Dad's not really strong, he likes to think he is, he's always squaring up to me for a box. Don't fancy his chances. Mind you, he has other ways of showing who's boss – you don't have to be all brawn."

"Look at old Jones. He's a wizard at maths and no one puts a finger out of place in his class and he's only two jampots high."

"Did you see Lambert at P.E. yesterday, he lifted Ben right over the box – one hand. He must be really fit, he always does cross-country with his classes and he comes in looking as though he'd been for a walk round the garden."

"We went to a wrestling match on holiday. Some of those fellows are all muscle – bulging out on their arms and chest."

15

"Well they train, don't they?"

"I reckon people only take notice of you if you look tough like that."

"Not really, it's more a quality in you – something people respect. The fellow who runs our club, he's a quiet gentle sort of person, yet when he says something has to be done, everyone listens and no one argues with him."

"All a matter of personality – bet you can't jump down without the rope."

Some did, some didn't.

*　　　*　　　*

Hormones .

That's what growing up is all about. Some can, some can't. Some are tough and big and strong – some are short and thin and wiry. In the end everyone reaches their maximum whatever that is and just as long as you accept yourself, so will everyone else accept you.

Whilst all this competition of muscle and strength is going on there are many unseen, unfelt changes happening inside these boys. Perhaps you're changing, too.

To understand these changes we must first know about glands and hormones. Hormones are special chemicals produced by special glands in the body. There are many different kinds of glands which produce special fluids to help the proper working of the body. They are very important. It is glands that make tears which can wash unwanted dust out of your eyes. Other kinds of glands keep your mouth moist and enable you to swallow.

You recall reading in the first chapter that the organs of your body are the same as those in a girl's, except for the sex organs. So it is with the glands. All these are the same in men and women – except for the sex glands.

You have two sex glands and they are called testicles. If you look back at the diagram on page 12 you can see them marked. They are inside the skin bag called the "scrotum".

They produce chemicals called hormones which enter the blood stream and circulate all through the body.

They also produce the life-cells from which new life is created. These are two important jobs for the sex glands to carry out in everybody.

Whereas the hormones work separately for each man and woman, the life-cells only make life when they join together. This is to say, no new life can be made unless the life-cell from a man is joined to the life-cell of a woman and so they become parents – the word means 'bringing to birth'.

That is why we normally have a father and a mother to care for us.

Each sex gland regularly gives out these chemicals called 'hormones' which enter the blood stream and so circulate all through the body. The male sex gland – the testicles – produces a chemical called testosterone.

This is what gives a man his 'manly' appearance. When you were a little boy you were not very different from the little girls you played with.

You had a high-pitched voice and a slim little body, and if your hair grew long, people often made a mistake and thought you were a little girl. Similarly people often mistake little girls for little boys, especially as so many wear jeans nowadays.

Well now that you are growing up becoming an adolescent — all that will change. The male sex gland begins to work and testosterone is released into your blood stream.

Your voice will 'break' and gradually become deeper. Hair will start to grow under your arms, on your chest and around your sex organs. Your shoulders will gradually grow broader and your muscles more pronounced.

The second function of the testicles is to produce the 'life-cells': the proper name for these is spermatozoa, which is often shortened to 'sperm'.

These sperms are very small, quite invisible to the human eye. They have little tails which enable them to move in fluid quite fast – something like a tadpole moving in water, but so small you cannot possible see them without the aid of a very powerful microscope, which is how doctors learn about these things. A fully developed man produces millions of these sperm continually.

If you look at this drawing of a sperm, you will see its 'head', called the 'nucleus'. This contains the hereditary parts of the life-cells, the features that are passed down the family. For instance, if your Dad is

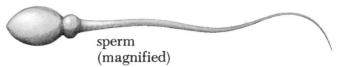

sperm
(magnified)

tall and dark there will be a tiny unit inside the sperm which could determine that a baby grown from this particular seed will be tall and dark. By itself, the sperm does not make a baby: it must be joined to the ovum or 'egg' produced inside a woman. The woman's egg also has a nucleus with hereditary parts, so you will have inherited some features from your father and some from your mother. If you look at your friends and their parents you will see how true this is.

3

"It makes me sick the way girls get away with everything."

"Me too. I only have to put a finger on my sister and Mum says, 'Remember she's only a girl,' and Dad says, 'Lay off her, you don't fight girls'."

"They want all the special treatment, but it's always their fault the row begins in the first place."

"Another thing, I don't see why I should do things like washing up when there are enough women in the house to do it."

"I agree, housework is a girl's job."

"My dad says it's shared. He always does some of the jobs in the house."

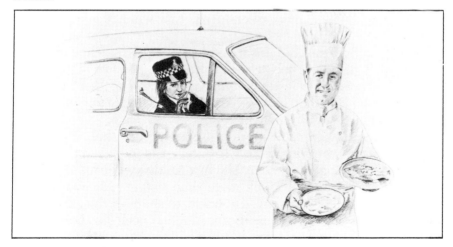

"Well he's married. It'll be different when we're married, I expect we'll have to help them."

"Well I shan't. I don't mind doing repair jobs and decorating and making things, but you won't catch me doing women's jobs."

"Suppose you like cooking? I mean, some of the world's best chefs are men!"

"Yes, and dress designers."

"And hairdressers."

"Well you don't see women building houses or making roads."

"You do in some countries, perhaps it's just our society that thinks there's a difference."

"Well I don't think there is any difference. When it comes to decisions and working it all out my Mum has just as much say as my Dad."

*   *   *

And so the discussion goes on. So it always will, because the roles and parts played by men and women are always changing and developing to suit the times in which they live.

Everything said here by the boys has been true at some time or is true now, or will be for them in the future.

Many years ago, in the time of early man, it was very easy to see the distinction between the roles of men and women. Men hunted, fought and protected the homes they had built. Women kept the homes clean, cooked and had children. Life went to a very simple pattern.

Today mothers and fathers are educated equally. They are both very capable people. They need to fulfil themselves in many ways. They both have basic instinctive needs which lead them towards being parents. But they also have other needs and want to achieve success in their own interests.

Marriage today is much more of a partnership than it has ever been. A mother wants to help contribute to the money in the home, to planning, buying, decorating and furnishing it. The man wants to share in the parenthood much more than before. He wants to be there at the birth of his baby. He wants to share in the caring and upbringing of the children. Both parents need to be equally important and necessary to each other and to the children.

It is possible to be equal to another person and yet different from him or her. It is the 'different from' that enables people to be attracted to one another.

You are attracted to your friends not only because you share some of their likes and dislikes but also because they are different from you. Everyone is unique and because of this you can find friends who answer your needs and share your fun and your moods with you. You become a good friend to them in the same way.

Sexual Attraction

The friendship which draws girls and boys, men and women together has the added bonus of 'sexual attraction'. You have learnt how hormones make men manly in a chemical way. Other hormones make women 'feminine'. There is a special attraction in this which

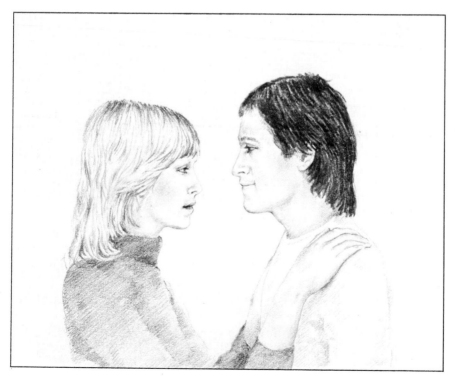

21

draws man and woman together and feeds their feelings for one another. What begins as friendship can turn to 'falling' in love' and then in marriage to a deep 'loving' of one another.

All this is not by accident or coincidence. It is designed in our nature so that man and woman want to love one another. They choose to get married and they want to have children of their own.

If all that was not natural and enjoyable, the whole human race would have ground to a halt thousands of years ago. Choosing to get married and wanting to have babies are two of the things which mark us out as different from all other living creatures. Many people today like to talk as though men and women are just a superior kind of animal. They forget how important the idea of 'free will' or 'free choice' is to human beings.

Animals can only 'mate' by instinct and they have no idea how their young are reproduced. It just 'happens' for them.

Human beings spend time deciding whether they will marry, and who they will marry. It becomes a decision of two thinking people. Then they may choose to have children, express their desire for children, and actually understand how to go about this and how the children are born.

This wonderful understanding that is special to men and women has to have some way by which a man or woman can learn to make the right decision. This 'responsibility' is one of the things which this book is all about. It is also one of the things which your parents, teachers and friends are most keen for you to learn and understand.

You—and other people

Anyone can look up information about how babies are born and how your bodies work. There are plenty of medical and scientific books to explain this. What your parents and those who look after you are hoping you will learn is not just the 'facts' but all the responsibilities that go with them.

They want you to understand as you grow up that 'sex' is not just a thing of the body, but a growing awareness of the 'other person', a growing love for people and eventually for one special person.

22

You wish to reassure them in these matters. It is not easy because you are still in that in-between stage of adolescence (the word means 'becoming adult'). You are so aware of yourself and your needs, it is difficult for you to think about the needs of other people.

Nevertheless, this is what growing up means. You make a choice. Either you remain like a child, always dependent upon your parents and making no decision for yourself, or you make the step forward to independence and becoming adult.

If you become adult still thinking only about what you want, you become a completely selfish person. Few people will want you for a friend, let alone marry you. But if you can try now at this stage to think how you affect other people, then you are on the way to becoming a lovable and loving person.

All this learning is much slower and harder to achieve than your physical change.

For instance, a young boy does not produce sperm. Sometime round about thirteen or fourteen or even later – there is no rule – the testicles will begin to produce sperm. It will happen quite suddenly and unexpectedly, and then the boy will become more aware of his change from child to man.

But this is only the physical sign – it does not change the 'person'. That is something slower and gradual—and much more difficult because you have to work on it youself. The physical happening you can do nothing about: you cannot stop it or start it. But the growth within yourself is your responsibility: you can help it or ignore it. Whichever you do, it is your decision. Parents and teachers and friends will all help (and sometimes hinder you), but the hard work of becoming the sort of man you want to be depends on you.

Listen to the boys talking about this very thing in the next chapter.

4

"I missed the school bus today."

"Unlucky you—did you get a detention?"

"Of course. But that wasn't all, I'd forgotten my maths book. In fact everything went wrong. When I got home I realised I'd forgotten to pick up the bread Mum asked me to get."

"A bit of a forgetful day you might say."

"It's all very well laughing about it, but everyone got in such a mood. I couldn't even settle down to my homework, so I just came out. Now I expect I'll get into another row when I get home for stamping out!"

"I get everything ready the night before and make notes about things I have to remember, otherwise I'd always be forgetting."

"You sound like my mother—she's always telling me to get organized."

"Well at least it keeps me out of detention."

"Oh sure, you're perfect of course."

"No need to take it out of me. I've got my own problems. You want to try living with my brother. He really stirs it for me. We have to share a bedroom and he occupies about four-fifths of it and I have what's left. His things are all over the place. I get told off all the time for being untidy. Just because he goes to work no one says anything."

"Well money makes a difference. It gives you independence."

"O.K., but it doesn't give you the right to use other people. He should still do his share in the family."

*　　*　　*

Those moods and situations happen to most young boys growing up. If you think about what they are saying, you will see that there are some things which they must take responsibility for—accept the consequences. Other things are not under their control, and then they must learn patience and tolerance.

At least they seem quite clear about independence. It has to be gained without cost to other people. It is the prize which comes when you have played the game properly without cheating the rules.

It is helpful, to begin with, if you can get rid of the idea that 'independence' is a declaration of war. All normal parents want you to have this: they know it is necessary as part of growing up for they have had to achieve it themselves.

Independence is a declaration about security. It shows a faith in your relationship with your parents. It says, 'we have enough going between us, in friendship and love, to enable me to take different attitudes from you without losing your affection and trust.'

They are continually on the look-out for signs of this maturity developing in you. They want you to be able to make decisions for yourself and to act in an unselfish manner towards family situations. Most of all, they want you to accept them as they are, for what they are is all they have been able to give you since the day you were born. (Stop and think about that for a minute.)

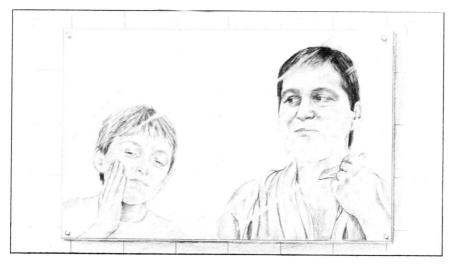

Adolescence—the facts

All this is part of the stage called adolescence. Everyone has been an adolescent before becoming adult: it is as natural as blossom to a tree—there is no fruit without it.

During this time your body is preparing for manhood, but you do not feel these changes like you feel moods. However, there are signs for you to recognize.

When the testicles start releasing the male hormones, your body will take on a new appearance. The muscles grow firmer and your limbs are stronger. Your shoulders broaden and your waist and hips are slimmer. The hair – called pubic hair – begins to grow under the armpits and against the pubic bone around the penis. At the same time hair begins to grow on the chest, and it darkens and thickens on the arms and legs. You may also notice the beginning of a beard, although this sometimes happens later.

Your voice drops in tone – people call this 'breaking'. The change in your voice can be quite gradual and may sometimes sound jerky. Some words came out in the high voice of a young boy and then suddenly drop to a low key. It can be embarrassing to you if you worry about this: you must just accept that it has happened to every man at some time.

Families often tease young people about these changes and draw attention to how 'tall', 'handsome', 'manly', etc. you are becoming. It is all well-meant since every family takes pride in its young people growing up.

There is also a change in your penis which becomes thicker and the testicles in the scrotum become firmer and a little larger. That prepares them for the next task which is to produce 'sperm' or life cells.

Once the sperms are produced they cannot be stored so they have to make their way out of the body by means of the penis. To make this easy a fluid is made by the seminal vessel and the prostate gland. Both these small organs swell slightly when the fluid is ready, then by contracting like a muscle, they squeeze the liquid out over the sperms which have travelled along the sperm tube.

You can see from the next diagram, how the sperms travel along the tube and past the seminal vessel and prostate gland, picking up the milky fluid on the way, and then into the urethra and out at the tip of the penis.

When the sperm and the fluid are mixed it is called 'semen'.

Male sex organs
(front view)

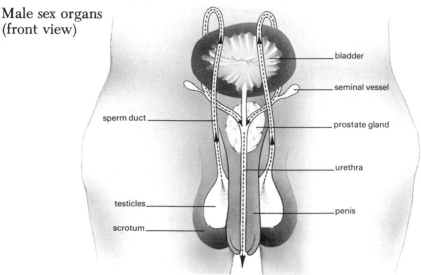

- bladder
- seminal vessel
- prostate gland
- urethra
- penis

sperm duct

testicles

scrotum

Most of the time you pass only urine through your penis, but at the times when semen is passed, the bladder is closed off from the urethra and only the semen passes out. This is called ejaculation.

Your first ejaculation will most probably happen when you are asleep. You cannot control it and therefore it is useless to worry about it. There is no magic age or date for this to happen. Some boys of twelve have ejaculations, some are fifteen or sixteen before it happens. But happen it does to all normal men.

Usually it happens in a kind of 'dream' whilst you sleep and this is why boys frequently call them 'wet dreams'. You may not even wake up, but if you do you will realise that your pyjamas or sheet are sticky wet, with a thickish white liquid. It is perfectly clean and harmless.

Do not be shy of telling your mother if you want the sheet cleaned or the pyjamas – she knows all about this. On the other hand it is one of these little matters in which you can show your independence by just rinsing the pyjama trousers yourself.

Wet dreams or ejaculations are another signpost you pass on the way to manhood. There is no way you can put the clock back. But there is still a lot of learning to do before you are 'in charge' of yourself. There is much to learn about responsibility and how to manage your sexual life in a sensible and caring way.

Earlier in this book you read about 'erections', and how they come about by the flow of blood to the tissues of the penis. This causes the penis to become firm and upright, instead of hanging limply between the legs. Sometimes this happens in quite small boys, but if it has not happened to you in childhood, it will certainly happen during this time of adolescence. It is only when the penis is erect that the semen can pass out so you will certainly experience erections when you have wet dreams.

Male sex organs
(side view)

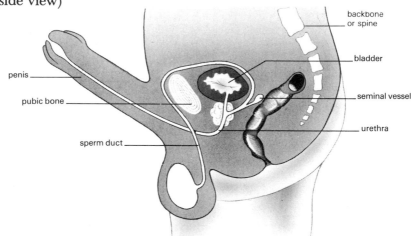

Sometimes you may find you get an erection during the daytime and you become very self-conscious about this uncomfortable situation. The quickest way to make it 'soft' again is to think hard about something totally different, a lesson or a television programme, or some job you have to do at the weekend and then it will become limp.

The important thing about all these happenings is that they are normal and necessary if you are to grow into a happy healthy man.

5

Andy, Nick, Pete and Tony are sitting on a bench in the middle of the shopping centre. One of their favourite pastimes these summer days is watching the 'talent' go by.

A few girls had already passed with knowing looks and backward glances, but no words were exchanged.

"What do you think girls talk about when they go around like that?"

"Same as us I suppose, talk about what they're going to do and who they saw and so on."

"You take just now for instance. I liked the little dark one with short hair and earrings—do you reckon they look at us and think he's good looking or he'd be alright to go out with?"

"More likely they're doing a cash count —girls only like boys who can take them out and give them a good time."

"I don't agree, some girls pay their share all the time."

"Pete's girl gives him presents, doesn't she, Pete?"

"So what. I give her things too. It doesn't mean anything."

"Why give presents if it doesn't mean anything?"

"Well I suppose it does mean something. You only give things to people you like. But it isn't serious."

"My Mum always thinks you're getting engaged or something when you give presents."

"Well that's how it used to be."

"I wonder what it's like being a girl, all the bother of periods and having babies—I wouldn't want to look forward to all that."

"What do you mean, 'periods'?"

"Don't you know anything?"

"Not about girls, we haven't got any in our family."

"That reminds me, you know those letters we had to take home from school about the sex film?"

"Yes, my mother says she can't see the point of it in school, she can tell us anything we want to know."

"Well you're lucky, my mum gets in a terrible state if I ask her anything about sex. She even gets embarrassed when the telly has plays about it. I'm glad we're going to see a film."

"I've seen it already in primary school. There's nothing in it—all diagrams and long words."

"Well perhaps the words won't be so long now. Anyway it'll be good for a laugh with old Jenkins. I bet he starts off with 'Now, boys, I want you to be very serious about this'."

And so the Saturday afternoon passed in laughs and chats and nods and winks.

*   *   *

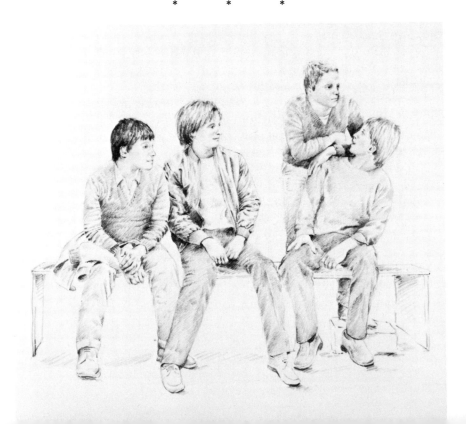

Many boys your age think and talk to each other about girls. They wonder about how they are made and they see the changes in them. They are attracted by them and at the same time nervous and anxious about how to relate with them. This is natural in a young adolescent and only time will reassure them. It is the same for a young girl—she is curious and interested, but also a little scared about getting involved in a friendship.

Because of this they both appear to do quite a lot of watching and waiting. They go to clubs and discos, or for walks in groups, but they nearly always stay with their own friends.

When the boys were talking together about girls, they were also looking for some answers about the sexual development of girls. They have already noticed that some adults find it easy to talk about these things whilst others find it embarrassing and difficult. One of the reasons why your parents gave you this book is to help you to become 'at ease' with the subject. They want you to be properly informed and to be able in your turn to pass the right information and the right attitudes to young people you meet and talk to.

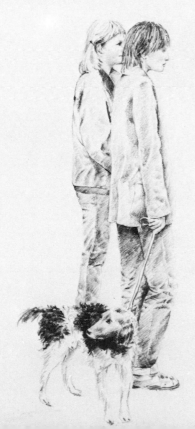

Over the last two or three years you have probably learnt some things about girls and how they grow up and also some ideas about babies and how they are born.

Girls ask about these things at quite an early age because it is about themselves and their own future, and they feel a need to know.

Boys do not feel so involved and so they may be less inclined to ask questions. The facts which they pass on to each other are often not complete and sometimes not correct.

Girls growing up—the facts

This section of the book will help you to get the facts you already know into some kind of order and will fill in any details that you are not sure about.

The drawing you see here is that of a female figure. Compared with the drawing you have of a man, there are some very obvious

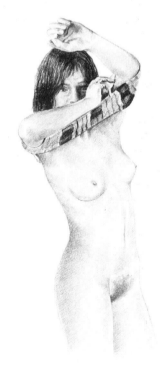

differences. A woman has breasts where a man is flat chested. The rest of her body is smooth and curved; she has no sexual organs outside of her body, as does a man.

Young children find this curious and little girls often talk about 'when my penis grows'. Sometimes they try to pass water standing up like their brothers – usually with uncomfortable results. However, by now you have accepted these differences but perhaps not thought about why.

It is a very simple answer. It is the woman who carries the unborn baby inside her for nine months. Therefore all the parts to do with having babies must be placed in the safest possible part of her. They are well protected by the back-bone and the pelvic girdle, and are deep inside her abdomen ('tummy').

Here is a diagram of these parts. If you could look with x-ray eyes, this is how the inside of a woman would look.

Some of the parts are just the same as in a man. If you compare the two diagrams you will see that both have a spinal column, a pubic bone, a bladder, a bowel and an anus. All these parts do exactly the same work for both male and female.

Female sex organs
(side view)

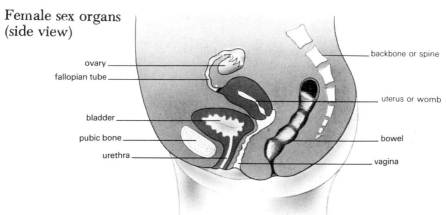

ovary
fallopian tube
bladder
pubic bone
urethra

backbone or spine
uterus or womb
bowel
vagina

The organs which are different are the sexual organs. You will remember that sexual means the nature of a man or a woman. The sexual organs are the parts concerned with reproducing life. The words 'sexual' and 'sexuality', however, have a much wider meaning for human beings than just reproduction.

33

The sexuality of a man is to do with his whole self and how he makes other people feel about him and also how he feels about himself. Although you are young you are already aware of some of these feelings. You enjoy feeling 'man-to-man' with your father. You feel 'gentle' towards your mother.

A girl also has sexual feelings at the same age. She feels womanly and motherly like her mother, she feels admired and pretty with her father. These are good feelings which come from happy families and help the young people to enjoy their growing sexuality.

Look again at the diagram on page 33 and find these parts:

The uterus (or womb)
The fallopian tube
The ovary
The vagina

Now look at the next diagram which shows a front view of the sex organs of a woman. Here you can see them quite clearly without all the surrounding organs and bones.

Female sex organs
(front view)

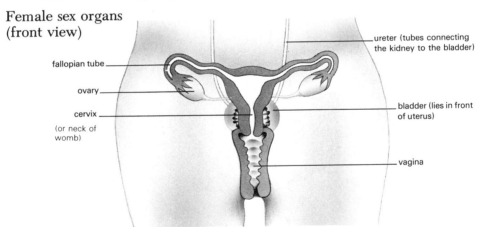

ureter (tubes connecting the kidney to the bladder)

fallopian tube

ovary

cervix

(or neck of womb)

bladder (lies in front of uterus)

vagina

As you read about these organs and how they work, look back to the diagram, find each name and see where it is.

The uterus is the Latin word for the womb. It is still used by doctors and medical books, but your mother would probably use the word 'womb'. This is a pear-shaped pouch with strong muscular walls which can stretch and shrink. It is inside this womb that a baby grows before it is born. That is why the walls have to be strong and able to stretch. After the baby is born the womb has to shrink back to its normal size of about three inches across.

The fallopian tubes: There are two of them, one on the right of the womb and one on the left. They reach from the ovary to the inside of the womb. They are the passages down which the ovum (egg) travels from the ovary into the womb.

The ovaries are situated one on either side of the womb, just at the ends of the fallopian tubes. They are the female sex glands. If you turn back to page 16 you can read again how important glands are in our bodies.

The sex glands in a woman, like those in a man, have two jobs to do. One job is to manufacture hormones and send them into the blood stream to circulate all through the body.

The hormones made by the ovaries are oestrogen and progesterone. The oestrogen gives the woman her 'womanliness'. It is produced at the start of a girl's adolescence. Because of this hormone she begins to grow breasts and her sex organs get larger. Hair grows under the armpits and in the pubic area around the vagina.

The progesterone is necessary to prepare the womb for a baby to live in.

The other job for the ovaries is to make the eggs ('ova': the singular is 'ovum') which are the life-cells from which a new life can be made.

The vagina is the passage from the lower end of the womb to the outside of the body between the legs. Everything that comes from the womb must come this way out through the vagina. The vagina, like the womb, has to have strong walls which stretch so that a baby can come this way into the world.

Now that you have found each of these organs and read what they are for, you can follow the next section which tells how they work in a woman.

You recall that at some time – you can't tell when – your sex organs begin to work and to make sperm. In the same way there is a time for the sex organs in a growing girl to start making ova (eggs). Girls begin adolescence at a younger age than boys, any time after twelve years of age—sometimes before then, but we have no way of telling just when it will happen. For boys and for girls, the body has its own 'built in' time clock which sets off the process of adolescence. It is all to do with the 'pituitary' gland, situated at the base of the head. It sends the message to the body that it is time for the sex organs to start their work.

You have already read what happens in a boy when this starts. In a girl it happens like this. One of the ovaries produces an egg. This is too tiny to see with the eye—it can only be seen with a microscope. At the end of the fallopian tubes are tiny fluttering ends like fingers which catch at the egg and draw it into the tube. It then travels down this tube into the womb.

If, on its journey, it does not meet any sperm to fertilise it, the egg will die within twenty-four hours. Farther on in this book you will read how the egg is fertilised – the word is used here to express what happens when the egg becomes a living cell capable of growing into a baby.

However, at this moment you are reading what happens at the beginning of a girl's adolescence, before she embarks on such a serious responsibility as having a baby.

At the same time that the egg is released the hormone called progesterone starts its work (you read about it a few pages back). It enables the womb to grow a soft lining to its walls. This lining is only needed when the egg is fertilised—it provides a place for the egg to become embedded and grow.

Since, in this case, it is not needed, that lining will come away from the sides of the womb and out through the vagina with a small loss of blood. This loss of blood lasts about five days and is called menstruation.

Girls call this their 'period'. During the time that a girl is having a period she wears a little cotton wool pad called a sanitary towel between her legs, inside her pants, to keep her clothing from being stained.

The journey of the unfertilised egg

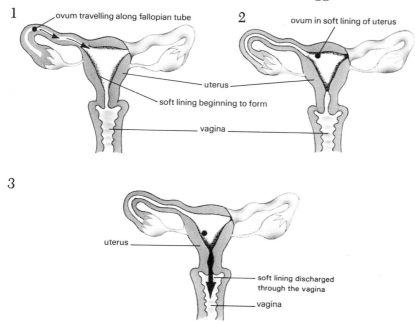

1 — ovum travelling along fallopian tube

uterus

soft lining beginning to form

vagina

2 — ovum in soft lining of uterus

uterus

vagina

3

uterus

soft lining discharged through the vagina

vagina

Although this is not an illness, it does sometimes affect the mood of girls. You may even have noticed with your own mother or sister that there are times when she seems more tired or more impatient with you. You may have said to your friends, "My mum is in one of her moods." This may just be the time when she is having a period.

Because you are growing up and becoming a man, you should be aware of these changes in people and be understanding and kind. Some day you may have a wife and she will really appreciate you if you show her kindness at such times.

6

"You going away for the holidays?"

"No, we can't afford it this year. Dad says we'll go out for days and have a good time."

"We're going camping by the sea. We go every year. They have a terrific time in these seaside camps. All the families go together – masses of aunts, uncles and cousins, and they *really* know how to enjoy themselves."

"I'm going to my married sister, Sue."

"That sounds a bore, I can't think of anything worse than a holiday with my sister."

"She's alright. She's not that much older than me so we get on very well. I like Chris—the man she's married to. He's good fun—it's more like staying with friends, going to them. Besides, Chris goes fishing with me and we stay out all night and have a really good time."

"Don't tell us you're an uncle!"

"Well as a matter of fact, I shall be soon, they're having a baby at Christmas."

They all fooled about, laughing at the idea of Andy being an uncle.

"Here, you know that film we saw about sex? D'you reckon that's what they do – to get a baby?"

"Do what?"

"Making love and all that, you see it all on telly."

"I expect it's different when you're married. I mean half the people on telly aren't even married and they don't have to think

about having a baby because it's just a play."
"In real life it would be serious, wouldn't it?"

Life together

Falling in love, making love, having babies—it's all a bit of a mystery to boys.

When you are young you are not really bothered about choosing a wife or being a father. You are still learning about yourself: only later on do you want to find out how to enjoy a girl's friendship without getting too involved.

Watching plays and reading books about sex, and talking together about these things are quite usual among growing boys. It is natural for you to be curious and to be a little anxious about experiences.

Older boys may tell you how they behave with girls and you may even sometimes think you are not normal or missing out on something if you are not having a great time with the girls.

Well, here's something for you to think about. Not all boys of your age want to go out with girls. If you're not interested at the present time, it doesn't matter: the day comes for everyone eventually. Lots of the talk you hear is just boasting and showing off. Boys are just as shy as girls about making friends.

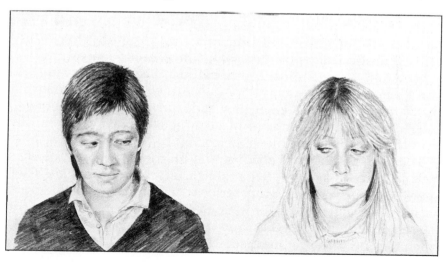

If you wish to be liked (and we all do) you must behave in a likeable way. This means putting the other person first. Whenever you are with a girl your intention should be to treat her in a way which makes her feel valued by you. Your respect for her will tell you how to behave. If she doesn't make you feel that you want to respect her, then she is not going to be a real friend.

Every good friend you make is a lesson in loving. You learn from friendships how to care, how to share, how to be tolerant and forgiving. Our families help us to learn this also, but it is a more difficult lesson in the family because it is so hard to start again after a mistake. In a family you are always you and most things you do get remembered too long.

With friends we change as we grow up. We start again and again, trying out different attitudes and styles, and each new friend accepts the way we are.

All that is very important and necessary because it leads eventually to choosing the right partner to live with for the rest of our lives.

Take Sue and Chris for instance, Andy's sister and brother-in-law. When Chris first met Sue he just thought she was a nice girl. She was quite pretty and good fun to go out with. They met for various 'dates' like discos and films. As they got to know each other better they relaxed more. Their talk became more natural. They were not afraid to disagree or have an argument. They could give in to each other.

The friendship deepened. As it grew deeper they grew closer together; not just closer in their interests, but physically closer. They enjoyed the 'feel' of being close, of holding hands, and kissing.

Soon they wanted to be together all the time, every parting was hard to make and they longed for the next meeting. When they put their arms around each other they had a great longing to belong to each other, to 'give' themselves in a new and different way from any kind of loving they had known before.

Then they began to talk about getting married, not a hasty careless 'let's get married at once', but a thoughtful, careful planning. They knew that marriage was a very serious decision. It is something you decide about and prepare for with great care. It is meant to last for the rest of your lives together, and that is what most couples intend when they decide to get married.

40

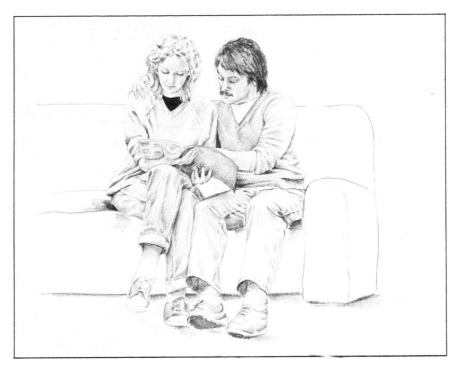

So Sue and Chris talked about a home, talked about children, talked about jobs and money. They spent evenings together making plans and learning about each other. It was all part of the preparation for a life together.

Eventually they decided to commit themselves to each other. They were 'engaged' and the day came for them to be married. It was the beginning of a long journey together in search of a great happiness.

At first there were little difficulties and arguments as they learnt to live together. They had to practise patience and tolerence. They learnt understanding and forgiveness.

They also learnt to love one another in a very special way that is designed for a man and woman.

You have already seen how the sexual parts of a man are outside his body and those of a woman are inside. You can see from the two diagrams that they fit together like two pieces of a jig-saw that join together to make the right picture.

41

When the husband and wife are loving in this special way they like to be as close as possible. They want to feel their bodies touching, skin to skin, and the man's penis fits into the vagina of the woman and then they are so close that they are almost one person. That is what the closeness of marriage means, really 'making love'.

They are loving one another and at the same time making more love.

Another word for this is intercourse. That's a kind of 'clinical' word which a doctor might use. Sue and Chris, and most married people would talk about making love, rather than intercourse.

They enjoy this experience very much, it is one of the great pleasures built in our bodies − to enjoy sexual love. If it was not enjoyable it is doubtful whether the human race would have survived, because this is the only way in which people can make babies.

All the parts of the body that are concerned with sex are very sensitive to touch. A man and woman making love become involved and alive and sensitive to one another, and these feelings awaken a strong need to embrace and to complete their union in one great feeling of love.

Knowing about this sensitivity and this strong need is important to you now that you are growing up. It will help you to be careful in your friendships. You do not want to awaken strong needs for making love with every girl you meet. This is something special for someone very special. Sue and Chris thought it was worth waiting to be married for this, because they wanted to belong just to each other and no one else.

It is not easy to understand words like 'deep love' and 'married love'. It is hard to imagine how 'strong' such love can be. Here are some ideas to help you.

You may have seen little children hugging their dads or mums. They squeeze them so hard their little faces are all twisted with the effort and they say 'I could hug you to bits' or some such nonsense. They are looking for words to say what is too big for them to describe.

Mothers sometimes say to their little children 'you're so good I could eat you.' This is another nonsense but it's the same idea—that love is too great for words. It almost seems to say, 'I can't get close enough, I'd like to climb right inside and be part of you.' Which is exactly what married love is all about.

At first Sue and Chris were quite content building a home and learning about each other, but eventually they had enough love spilling over to want a baby to share this. So now Sue is 'pregnant', which means she has a baby growing inside her womb.

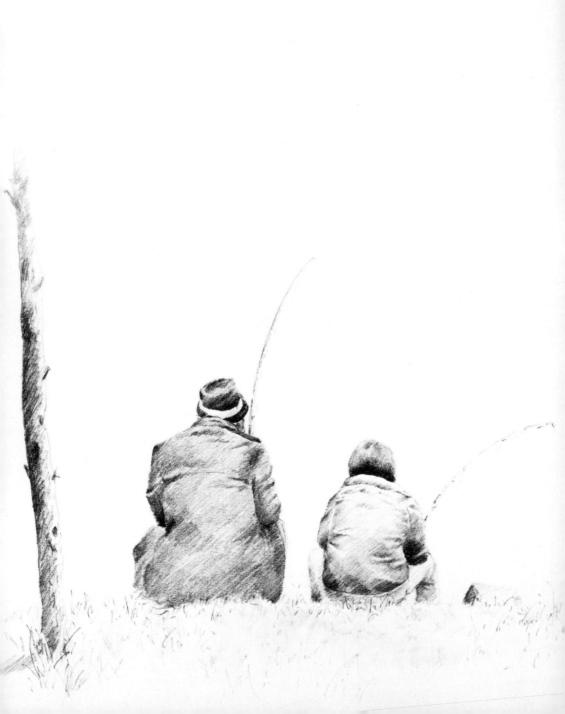

7

"Coming fishing tomorrow Chris?"

"I might, I haven't mentioned it to Sue yet."

"It's my last night here."

"I know, but I have to think about Sue, she might not like being left on her own at night. I'll let you know."

The following Saturday saw Chris and Andy well settled-in by the river bank with chairs, flasks, food and maggots.

"Sue didn't mind, did she? She's never minded before about you going fishing."

"It's different now, with the baby coming along."

"I can't see what difference that makes."

"Well it does. Girls change quite a lot when they are pregnant. They are more sensitive—you know, you have to be more gentle about how you talk to them. They like you to take care of them and spoil them a bit."

"Sounds a lot of fuss about nothing to me."

"That's because you're not married. When you get married it's not just "girls" any more, it's your wife you are talking about. She's much more special and worth giving a lot of attention to. After all it's our baby, not just hers. I want to be around as much as possible. If I can't have the baby at least I can make it a happy time for her. That's why I do more jobs in the home now."

"If you mean like getting a cup of tea in bed, I'm all for it, I salute the new Chris."

"You were just getting fringe benefit! It was Sue who woke up early and said she was thirsty."

"I can't imagine ever getting married. It sounds so serious and boring compared with my life. We have a great time, Tony, Pete and Nick and myself. No ties, free to go where we like, when we like, how on earth could you face giving all that up and getting tied down to one person? I mean Sue's alright, I suppose, even though she's my sister, but I can't think how anyone wants to get married."

"I know what you mean. I suppose I thought just like you at your age. But we don't stay still at any age, we keep on growing up. What you call "great" now will be boring for you in a few years. Then you'll want some other kind of goal in life.

"You get fed up in the end with just "girls". You begin to want a "steady" girl. One that you can relate with and be comfortable and not always wanting to "show off" to. That's how it was with Sue. After I'd been out a bit and came home and met you all, I just began to see how well we "fitted". Sue and I liked lots of things together and we enjoyed the same kind of laughs. We became "sure" of each other. I mean we didn't have to wonder any more about what each of us was doing or whether we still liked each other or if there was anyone else in the running. We just knew we were happiest together."

"But how can you be sure? Suppose you met someone else?"

"They're all questions that people ask before they decide to get married. Once you've decided you have to work on the idea together. You could spend all your life wondering if it was the right decision: then you'd find you'd missed out on all the good times, worrying about it. I just don't think about it any more. I enjoy what I have, it's a good life and we are glad we got married."

"If you heard the way some of the boys talk, you'd be surprised. They don't reckon being married is a good life — in fact some of them think it's pretty awful from what they've experienced."

"What's your experience? Do you reckon your mum and dad have been happy?"

"I suppose so, never thought about it much, perhaps I'm just lucky."

"There are plenty of 'lucky' ones as you call it. The reason you don't think about it is this: just because your home is normal and happy, you can take it for granted. The boys who don't want to marry because of their own unhappy families need to talk about it, they need support. You don't help them by agreeing with them, you have to share with them your *good* feelings about your family."

"I don't have any good feelings!"

"Come off it, Andy! You know you don't mean that. Every teenager has disagreements with his family. In fact the only reason you *can* blow your top at home is because you know you are absolutely safe—no one's going to turn you out or beat you up."

They surveyed the murky depths of the river in silence for a while.

"Chris."

"Hm."

"What do you think about masturbation?"

"I don't. What do you think about it?"

"Do you reckon it's wrong to masturbate?"

"Lots of boys do. But if you're asking me whether it's wrong, something or someone must have suggested to you it is wrong."

"Well, people don't exactly shout about it so there must be some reason for keeping it quiet, as if it's something you're not supposed to do."

"That's not a bad way of looking at it because it's usually only a passing phase; eventually you will come to the stage in your life when proper sexual intercourse will take its place.

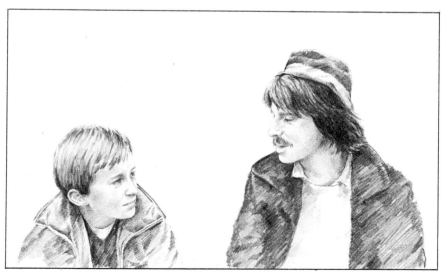

"It's a kind of 'comfort' thing. Little boys sometimes rub their penis in their sleep, or to get to sleep, because it is a pleasant sensation and makes them feel relaxed and comfortable. When they get older they sometimes do this to get an erection and get rid of some of their sperms. They don't have to get rid of sperm this way because "wet dreams" will look after that for them. But it is a nice sensation or feeling to do it yourself by rubbing your penis up and down with your hand. It is the same kind of pleasant feeling as you get with intercourse. I say intercourse because I can't call it making love. That has a special feel of its own. Making love is the physical pleasure plus the happiness of giving yourself to someone you love and receiving their love in return. That kind of loving is for two people and its direction is always away from you and towards someone else.

"When you masturbate it's like turning the feeling round so that it faces you. It doesn't go out anywhere: it just turns back into you, so that in the end it becomes yourself loving yourself. That is why boys have this mixed-up feeling that it is partly enjoyable and partly bad or wrong.

"We are brought up to believe that we should be unselfish and think of others and so anything that is completely self-centred and only for our own pleasure leaves us with a slightly guilty feeling and we don't want people to know."

"So you are saying that it is wrong?"

"I'm explaining why it "feels" wrong. You shouldn't worry about it because the desire to do this will pass as you grow older and manage your sexual feelings better. I used to have all these worries just like you but now I'm married I don't even think any more about it.

"If a boy decided this was the great way for getting pleasure and settled for it as his way of expressing sexual feelings—*that* would be wrong. But as long as he is aware that this is not the true or proper way of gaining sexual satisfaction, then eventually he will get himself sorted out and he won't need to masturbate."

"What about the boys who say sex is just an instinct like any other appetite? If you're hungry you eat so if you want sex why shouldn't you have it?"

"That's a description of an animal, not a human being. Animals do everything by instinct. The thing which makes us different and special is that we have a will to control our instincts. Growing up is very largely a matter of training our will. When we are young other people make that decision, we don't have much chance to use our own will. But once we are adult we have to be in charge of ourselves and choose how we behave. We have to use our will to make it happen the way our reason tells us is best.

"If you settle for anything less you're just an animal. It's the oldest con-trick in the book, Andy, telling you to obey your instincts. Use your intelligence instead and work out your own answers. Instincts are useful guides and send you messages, but they are not in charge of you."

A fish leapt at a fly making little rings in the water. Their thoughts floated out and away on the ripples and their concentration was all on the catch: the *instinct* of the hunter, harnessed to the *skill* of man.

8

"It's all very well telling us we'll grow out of it, but it's jolly embarrassing having spots all over my face."

"My sister gave me some special cream. She said you can get it at a chemist. It's not bad."

"Old Lambert seemed to think all you do is use hot and cold flannels and soap."

"He's so old he probably thinks acne is a form of rheumatism."

"Well I don't see how you get a girl when you've got spots all over your face."

"You wear a notice saying 'I've got acne, but I'll grow out of it'."

"Girls have it too, haven't you noticed the third-years?"

Hygiene

That little conversation could be heard in any group of young boys growing up. It is always an embarrassment and a worry to young people, boys or girls, how to cope with skin troubles.

What happens is that in adolescence when all these glands we have mentioned become active, there are also some changes in the sweat glands. You will find that you sweat much more after exercise than you did as a child. The sweat glands under the armpits and across the shoulders at the back become particularly active.

Another cause of sweating is nervousness or anxiety. Quite ordinary things that gave you no anxiety before will suddenly seem like huge problems that make you sweat just to think about them.

For instance, if you are asked a question in class, or if you have to make a journey on a bus alone or buy something in a shop, you can suddenly get an overwhelming feeling of embarrassment. You think all the class is looking at you, or everyone on the bus, or all the people in the shop are staring. These are quite common feelings among teenagers and they are perfectly normal. As 'Old Lambert' says, you grow out of it.

Sometimes the increased sweating causes a build up of grease under the skin and then if one of the little skin ducts get blocked you will get blackheads or rather angry looking spots called acne. Again you just have to be patient and wait for this to pass. But you can help yourself. Plenty of washing with clean hot water and flannels will certainly take out a lot of grease from your skin. You can pay a little attention to diet. Cut out some of the 'greasy' foods like chips and crisps, and increase the fresh fruit.

Exercise is tremendous for improving looks. It tones up your whole body, brings extra oxygen to your skin and brightens your eyes. In fact if you look at anyone coming in from a good brisk walk or an outdoor sport you will see that they 'glow'. So do not underestimate what you can do for yourself in the way of good looks.

It is also important to take showers frequently and if necessary use deodorants. There are plenty of toilet goods on the market for men, and an unlimited amount of aunts who never know what to get nephews for Christmas—so just put your favourite brand around.

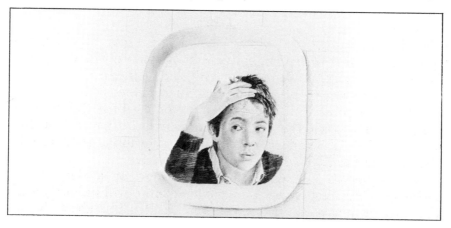

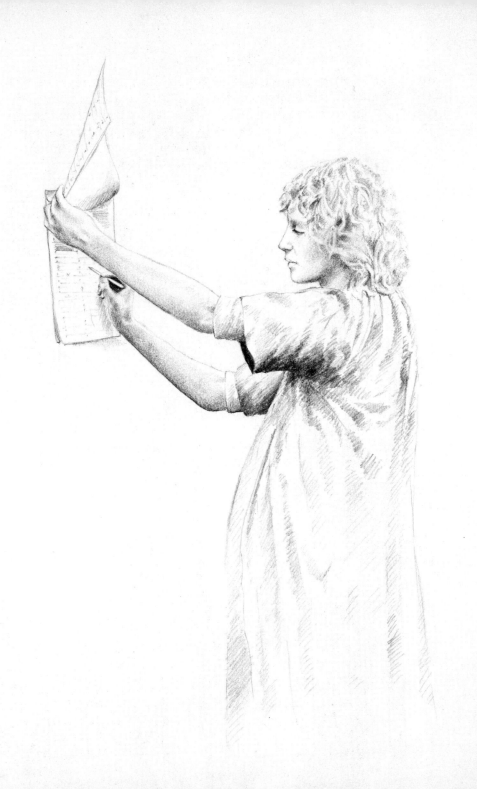

9

"Aren't you an uncle yet, Andy?"

"Get away—the baby isn't due until Christmas."

"It's a jolly long time since you told us Sue was having a baby."

"Only a few months ago. It takes nine months, you know."

"We have an expert here on the subject, boys."

"It must seem an awful long time for a girl to wait—nearly a year!"

"Sue said it goes quickly: there's such a lot to get ready."

"What I don't understand is how it actually happens. I mean I know we did some lessons on reproduction and saw that film, but I couldn't follow it all. I got lost in all the long names and diagrams, and I couldn't really follow the explanations."

"You could have asked last week when old Jenkins mentioned it for revision."

"Oh yes, and have everyone laugh at me. You know very well that everyone pretends they know it all because they don't want to be the one who asks."

"I ask Chris anything I want to know, he's easy to talk to. Why don't you ask Jenkins when he's on his own? He's quite decent to talk to."

How it actually happens

Nick is just like many boys of his age. He has some idea about how babies are made and born, but he would like some gaps filled in. He feels too old now to ask at home, so it's a good idea to find someone —

like Andy has — whom he can trust and depend on, and ask questions openly and frankly.

Here is a simple explanation to help you sort out what you already know, and perhaps add some extra information.

To understand how the baby is 'made' you will need to go back and look at the journey of the egg in the woman, and see how the sperm from the man is passed in a milky fluid out of his penis.

Usually, as you know, the penis is a soft fleshy thing which hangs down between the legs. You have also read how in adolescence it grows firmer and stronger. When the fleshy part is filled with blood, it becomes erect.

When a husband and wife are making love, the touching of each other and their caressing causes the erection and this enables the penis to slide firmly into the vagina. At the climax of their love-making, the penis, by means of a muscular movement, can send the semen into the vagina. This is called ejaculating.

The sperm can now travel alone by means of tiny propelling tails, through the womb and up into the fallopian tubes.

Here is a diagram of how the sperm makes that journey.

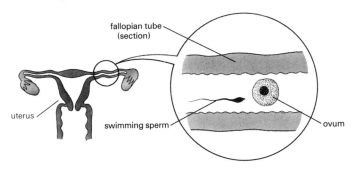

The picture is greatly enlarged to make it clear for you, but in actual fact the sperm is far too small to see with the eye.

The sperm can only live for about four days, so it is necessary, in order to make a baby, for the sperm to reach the tubes at the same time in the month that an ovum has been released from one of the ovaries.

If there is no ovum present, the sperm will simply die and pass out again through the vagina. If however, it is the right time in the month for the ovum to be released into the tubes, then the sperm will gather round this egg. The strongest sperm will force its way into the ovum and fertilise the egg.

This is what 'fertilise' means – making a life. Life can only be made by bringing the sperm and the ovum together. There is no way that an ovum or a sperm can make life on its own.

The pictures show you an ovum with the nucleus inside it and the sperm gathered around. The second picture shows how a sperm pushes its way into the ovum and the nucleus head of the sperm joins the nucleus of the ovum. Once that has happened a new life is on its way to being born.

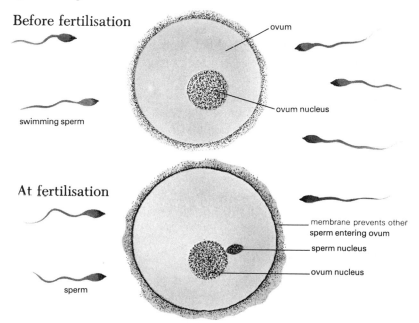

Before fertilisation

ovum

swimming sperm

ovum nucleus

At fertilisation

membrane prevents other sperm entering ovum

sperm nucleus

ovum nucleus

sperm

It is at this moment of fertilisation that a new life is begun. This is sometimes called 'conception'. The new life has been 'conceived'.

Nobody really understands how life is made. We know it happens when certain things are put together, like sperm and ovum, or earth and seed, but we don't know what the 'life' is that sets growth in motion. Not even the smallest blade of grass can be *made* to grow: it either does or does not—we have no power over this mystery.

This is why it is such a serious thing — this 'making a baby'. It is entering into the secret of creation.

You read in another chapter in the book how both the ovum and the sperm carry chromosomes which give the baby its characteristics. All that happens at exactly the same time as the fertilisation takes place. From the moment a new life is begun these chromosomes decide whether the baby will be a boy or a girl, tall or short, dark or fair and many other distinctive features that all go to make a unique person unlike any other in the world.

How the baby grows in the womb

The new life will grow in the mother's womb for nine months. In that time it has special care and nourishment to prepare it for the time of birth.

The fertilised egg will take about ten days to move down into the womb. You will recall that during this time the womb is preparing a lining, a special bed, in which the fertilised egg can bury itself and grow.

Here is a picture of the inside of the womb with the egg firmly planted in the lining. From now until the baby is born, the mother will have no more periods because there are no linings to shed. The hormones in the woman will change their work and so no more eggs

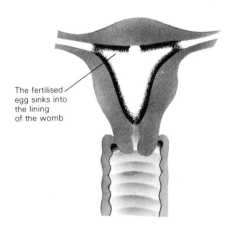

The fertilised egg sinks into the lining of the womb

will be sent out into the fallopian tubes whilst the mother is carrying her baby inside the womb.

After a month the little round egg begins to take the shape of a baby. It is no longer called an egg, but an 'embryo'.

The next picture shows you an embryo about six weeks old.

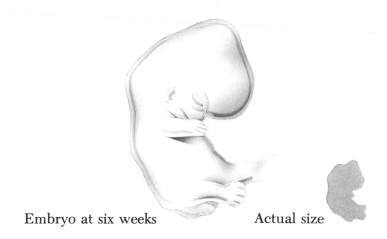

Embryo at six weeks   Actual size

This embryo is already ten thousand times bigger than the day it was conceived. So it is easily visible with the human eye.

Several new tissues and fluids have come into being with the embryo baby (look at the second diagram on page 59):

The protective fluid is a kind of warm water in which the embryo baby floats. It is a protection like a soft cushion. It stays with the baby right up till the time of birth. It is a protection from all the bumps and jolts of everyday life of the mother.

The placenta is very important indeed — the unborn baby cannot live without it. It is the source of food and oxygen for the baby.

The umbilical cord is a twisted stringy line of blood tissues joining the baby to the placenta. There are two blood vessels: one carries new blood to the baby and the other takes away the stale blood.

Everything the mother takes into her own blood stream will pass through the placenta and the cord to the baby. This is why it is important that a mother should eat and drink only what is good and nourishing for herself and the baby.

Smoking produces nicotine in the blood and alcohol also enters the blood stream, so mothers who are carrying babies should take great care not to damage their baby with these drugs or any form of strong medicine.

The whole of the nine months in which a mother is carrying her baby is called her 'pregnancy'. A pregnant woman means just this, a woman who is carrying, i.e. 'expecting', a baby.

By the third month the embryo becomes a 'foetus' and this word is used by doctors until the baby is born. In the next few weeks the heart and lungs and organs of a tiny human being are formed and begin to work. Doctors can hear the heart beat quite clearly and often allow mothers to listen to it, to reassure them.

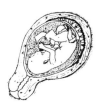

The foetus in the womb at 3 months old

By the end of four months the mother can feel the baby moving inside her. It is just like tiny feeble flutters at first, but gradually as the baby grows strong and bigger the movements are much more definite and the father, if he puts his hand on the mother's stomach, will feel the baby kicking and stretching. The top diagram opposite shows the baby after six months.

During the months of growing the baby will turn around many

58

The foetus in the womb at 6 months old

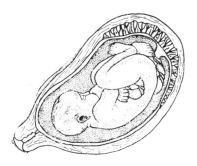

times and with ease. Towards the end of the nine months, however, the baby will remain head downwards and resting at the neck of the womb. This is the easiest position for the birth of the baby.
The baby is ready to be born

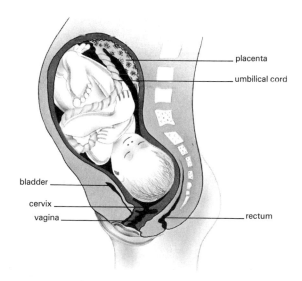

placenta

umbilical cord

bladder

cervix

vagina

rectum

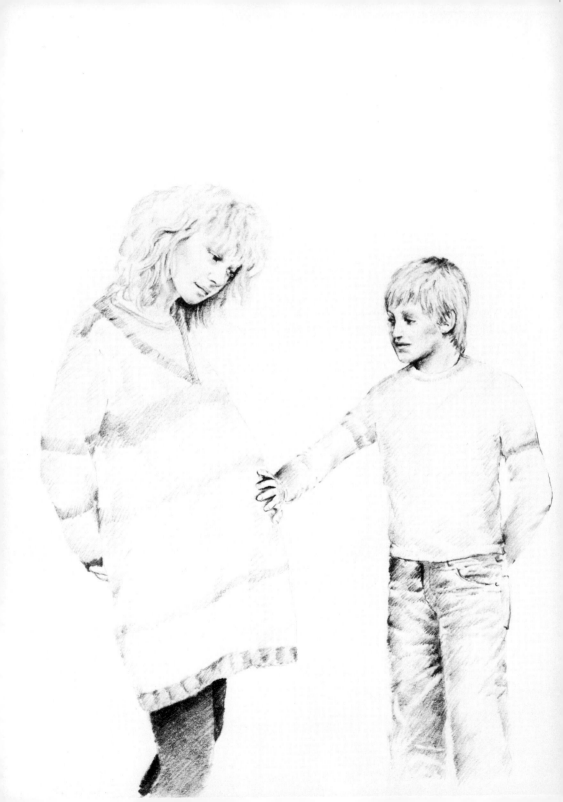

10

"You sit down and talk to Andy, I'll wash up," said Chris to Sue. Chris went out to the kitchen.

"Unbelievable, you must have magic power over Chris!", said Andy, amazed.

"He's been marvellous, he takes such good care of me I feel like royalty every day."

"You'd better make the most of it, he'll probably go back to normal when the baby arrives."

"I don't think so, he'll be so interested he'll want to help with everything. Even now he wants to know about the baby, how it feels and which way up it is, and everything."

"Can you tell?"

"I can certainly feel it. The little fellow never stops thumping me." There was a moment's pause.

"Sue?"

"Yes?"

"Nick said his mother once had a miscarriage. He was only young and all he remembers is doctors coming and going, and some aunt coming to look after him. But he says he can remember being told about a new baby brother or sister coming and then it never came. No one said anything more about it and he just waited and waited until he forgot all about it."

"Poor thing," said Sue. "He didn't understand and no one thought to tell him because he was so young. They couldn't have realised how a little boy would take in so much and want to know what was going on."

"Could it happen to you?"

"No, my baby is well established and the doctor at the clinic sees me regularly to make sure everything is in order.

"Just occasionally, a fertilised ovum doesn't get a proper fixing in the womb and so the womb gets rid of the embryo because it is imperfect. Or, maybe it starts to grow and then something goes wrong, so again the womb will reject it. Sometimes the reason is to do with the mother's health, or the blood group of one of the parents. There are lots of medical reasons why she may have a miscarriage and quite a lot of unknown reasons. Doctors are always studying these things and learning more about how to put them right."

"Is it the same as a 'premature' baby?"

"No. In the case of a miscarriage, there is no way the foetus can live. It hasn't developed sufficiently to have its own life. A miscarriage usually happens in the early months of pregnancy.

"But although a premature baby is born a few weeks before the full nine months are completed in the womb, the baby is sufficiently well-developed to live and the birth is usually normal. It just means that because the baby is so small it is not strong enough to live without special help to replace the extra time it should have had in the mother's womb.

"What usually happens is that the doctor places the baby in an incubator which is a specially heated little bed-tent that keeps the baby as nearly as possible in the same warmth and security as in the womb. After a few weeks the baby has grown strong enough to live normally and go home with its mother."

"I bet you wish you knew whether you were having a boy or girl!"

"Not really. It's part of the excitement, waiting to know. Besides, think how disappointing it would be if you really made up your mind you wanted a boy and then found out it was going to be a girl."

"I expect they'll discover some way of telling one day."

"They already have, but I don't want to know before the baby is born. Whatever my baby is, is already decided; nothing I can do will change that—and I am glad. I wouldn't want the responsibility of deciding."

"It might be twins. You might have a boy and girl at the same time—that would be a laugh!"

"It might be a laugh for you—it wouldn't be for me. I've only knitted one lot of everything!

"Anyway it isn't twins. The doctors can tell that sort of thing very early in the pregnancy and they would have told me by now."

"How do people get twins? Is it just luck?"

"Well they quite often run in families. We don't have any twins in our family or in Chris's so it's not very likely to happen to us.

"There are two kinds of twins – identical and non-identical.

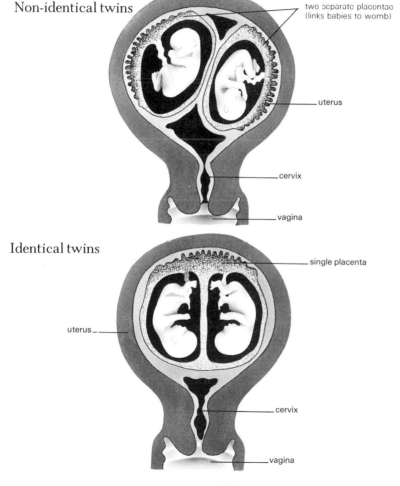

Non-identical twins

two separate placentae (links babies to womb)

uterus

cervix

vagina

Identical twins

single placenta

uterus

cervix

vagina

63

"If the ovum divides immediately after the sperm has fertilised it you have identical twins. They will be two boys or two girls, and they will look exactly alike. I'll draw you a picture so you can see what I mean.

"See how the babies float in separate sacs of fluid with separate cords but are attached to the same placenta?

"Now if by chance the ovary releases two eggs at the same time and both become fertilised, then you have non-identical twins. In that case they develop quite separately in the womb, each with its own placenta, like this."

Chris came in as Sue was explaining,

"Your little chat seems to have turned into quite a biology lesson," said Chris.

"It's very interesting. I wouldn't mind being a doctor and knowing all these things."

"Being a father is not a bad way of finding out!"

11

"Going to the end of term disco?"

"I expect so, though I don't know why, they're always a bore."

"Come off it! You enjoyed the last group we had."

"Oh the music's alright, it's just that nothing ever happens. All the boys congregate down one end and all the girls at the other. Sometimes the girls get up and dance, but never with the boys, they just stare at us and whisper and giggle."

"Hey, you've got a complex or something. We stare enough at them."

"You going to walk Kate home, Pete?"

"I might—she might not let me. Girls are funny, you can't tell if they don't like you or if they are just shy."

"I wouldn't know what to do if a girl said I could walk her home."

"You soon find out. Most girls let you know the sort of girl they are. You just play it cool and don't rush them."

"The voice of experience!"

"Well I've been around you know."

"Don't we know it! Your reputation gets around as well. You must have dated more girls than you've had school dinners."

"Well at least I keep them all happy. I don't collect broken hearts. There's no point in getting involved at our age. Girls are just experience, they teach you how to treat them. But I don't want to get tied down to one girl."

The right kind of friendship

Girls are always a bit of a problem to boys the age of Andy and his friends. Even if you have not yet had a date with a girl, you will be very aware of them and conscious that you are expected at some time to get interested in them.

Reading and understanding about how you are developing, and also how a girl grows up and matures, should give you some confidence. But mostly time and experience will be your teacher. You will be attracted to many different kinds of girls. You yourself will change your interests and needs as you grow older. The girls you choose as your friends will be right for a particular time in your life, but not necessarily for always.

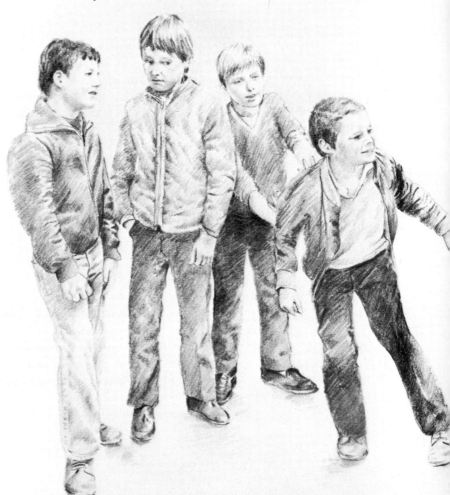

Choosing a partner for the rest of your life is a very serious decision and you don't want to be that serious now. It carries many responsibilities that you are not yet able to take on board.

Think about the sacrifices Chris makes for Sue, how he considers her first before going fishing or anywhere else. Look how he helps her in the home and shares in the preparation for the baby. They don't seem like a hardship to him because he is older and more mature than you are and wants to have these responsibilites. You are probably like Andy, still enjoying your freedom, enjoying your friends and taking in all the interests and new experiences that life offers you.

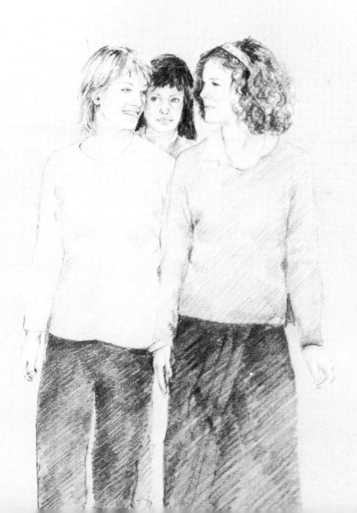

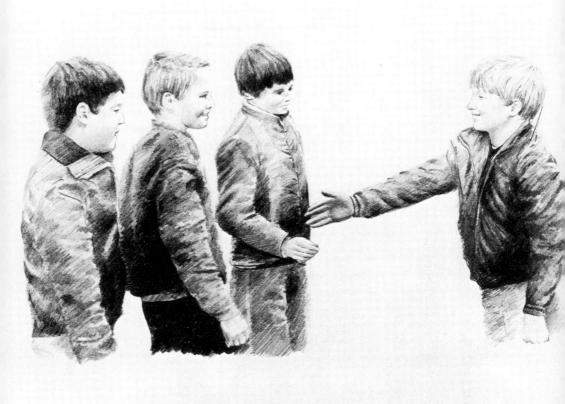

12

"Well, congratulate me, boys!"

"You're an uncle! Get that! Uncle Andy."

"When was the great day?"

"Last night as a matter of fact."

"Last night? I thought I saw Chris dropping you at the square last night."

"You did. That was earlier—he called in to leave some presents for Christmas."

"But didn't he know the baby was coming that night?"

"No, of course not. You can't tell in advance. When he got home Sue was icing the Christmas cake. She didn't go into the maternity home until nearly midnight."

"Crikey!"

*   *   *

Andy's friends were so surprised at the suddenness of birth that they actually became silent. A birth always comes as a surprise, even though we seem to be waiting for it. The moment of our coming is as unknown as the moment of our death. Even the mother shares a sense of awe and wonder when she looks at the new little person in her arms, so suddenly in this world after so long in the womb.

During the nine months the baby has lived in the womb it has become strong and well developed in every organ and limb. The time has come for it to make a separate life from the mother—to be born.

69

The baby being born

1

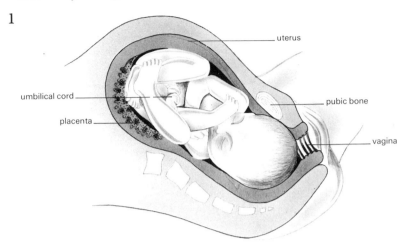

umbilical cord

placenta

uterus

pubic bone

vagina

2

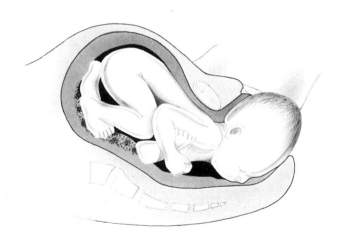

How the baby is born

Usually the mother has signs of this coming a few hours before the birth. The womb, which is like a large muscle, makes tightening and loosening movements to push the baby out. The sac of fluid breaks and the 'water' drains away through the vagina. The mother can feel the head of the baby, and the pushing becomes stronger and more urgent. She is compelled to push out the baby in a kind of rhythmic pattern, known as 'contractions'.

This is called 'labour'. There is a first stage which is slower and prepares the mother. Then there is a second stage which is much harder, but usually not so long. It is not comfortable or easy for the mother, but she can bear it because of the great excitement and the longing to have her baby in her arms.

The drawings opposite show you the stages of the baby as he is born. You can see his position in the womb and how the neck of the womb and the wall of the vagina must stretch and open to allow the baby through.

As soon as the baby appears, helped by a midwife or a doctor, the mother is told whether it is a little boy or girl.

Then the midwife gives a little sharp slap on the back of the baby to start him breathing. As soon as that happens the baby gives a loud wail and everyone is delighted because all is well and the little baby has announced his presence to all.

Now all that has to be done is to cut the baby loose from the cord which attaches it to the placenta. The cord is tied as firmly as possible close to the stomach and this will become the navel. You have this mark with you all your life.

About fifteen or twenty minutes after the baby is born the placenta will come away from the womb and pass out through the vagina with a little blood. The womb will continue for a few days to lose a little blood as it does in a period. After that it shrinks back to its original size of about three inches.

It is quite usual nowadays for fathers to be invited to be present at the birth of the baby. It is a great encouragement to the mother to have her husband with her and the moment of joy can be shared by both.

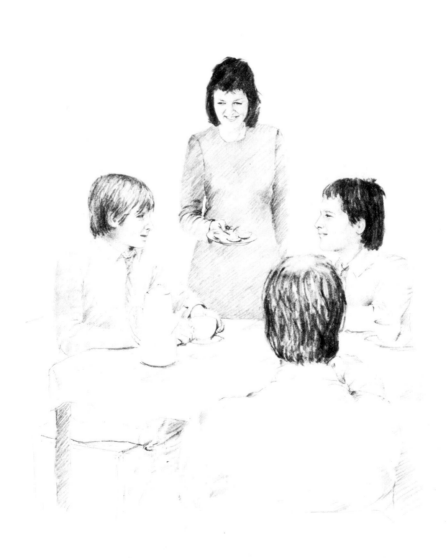

13

"So where were you when there was carol singing to be done?"

"Oh Lord, I forgot all about that! Did you collect at the station again?"

"Yes, it's the best place. It's easy to get to for everyone and there are plenty of people about."

"And they're in a generous mood on Christmas Eve so they don't mind giving something."

"Just as well, if you depended on the musical performance you wouldn't get much."

"Old J. was in a good mood this year, he asked us back to his house and we had coffee and mince pies. His wife's quite nice, not a bit like you'd think."

"How do you mean?"

"Well, you know, she's pretty and jolly and friendly. I never think of teachers as being just fathers or husbands in their homes. He seemed quite different and she talked to us just as though we were visitors. They've got three children, one's married and the other two live away from home. They were all coming up for Christmas though."

"We went to Sue and Chris because mum thought the journey here would be too much for Sue with such a new baby. That's how I forgot the carol singing; we went off on Christmas Eve."

"I got off to a bad start Christmas Eve—had a row with the old man. I said I thought it was a bore all this visiting and family round the telly and endless food. He gave me the usual lecture on family duties and my selfishness, so I went off without any supper saying I didn't care what he thought about me and I'd be glad when I could leave home and I wouldn't expect my kids to stay in over Christmas."

"I would. Anyway I don't know where people go if they don't have any family. No one wants other people when they've got a house full and everything is shut in the town."

"Yes, I know that really. I just suddenly thought I couldn't bear all the same talk and everything going on the same as always. But when we went back to Jenkins' place and I saw the tree and the house all ready for their family to come home, it seemed right really. That's where you have to be—at home. I even felt sorry for the old people we were collecting for. It's not much compensation is it—a few pounds and some tinned food instead of a family round you?"

"What's it like being an uncle, Andy?"

"Average, pretty average! He's ever so small. Unbelievable! When you hold him you think you're going to pick up a weight and he's as light as a feather. I reckon all the nappies and gear weigh more than he does."

"I'd like to have seen you giving him his bottle: what a laugh — 'come along children, drinkee time'."

"Idiot! Anyway, he doesn't have a bottle. Sue feeds him herself."

"Funny that, when you think about it, how a mother feeds her baby. I mean you don't usually think about that when you're looking at girls."

"You mean you don't!"

"Come off it. How many fellows look at a girl and say, 'she's got a nice pair, her baby will be lucky'?"

They all laughed. Andy said, "I know what you mean, I thought that too. When I saw Sue feeding young Mark it just looked so natural and the baby all cuddled up and enjoying it. It's quite a different way of thinking about things."

"If girls only have bosoms to feed babies, I don't see why they are so interesting to boys."

"Well, it's both, Chris says. It's part of what makes a girl 'sexy' but it also has a useful purpose like feeding a baby."

"What does a mother have to do to get milk there?"

"Nothing, Sue says. It just comes all of its own accord when the

74

baby is born. Something to do with hormones and glands and things. The more the baby drinks the more it comes back."

"A regular dairy, so to speak. Coming to club tonight?"

"Probably. You coming, Nick?"

"Might — the old lady kicks up a bit if I go out too often. Well, see you."

*   *   *

It's nearly a year since the boys sat in a tree talking about parents and freedom and the responsibility of growing up.

Perhaps you too have been through some of these stages with the boys. You may even feel that you know exactly how some of them talk about girls or families. Like the boys in this book, you have been able to sort out some of the knowledge you already have and also added some facts that were only questions before.

It is easy and quick to gain information about the facts of reproduction. Any good dictionary, together with a biology book, will give you this knowledge. It is a much slower and more difficult lesson to learn the facts about relationships. Learning about ourselves and then about how we are with other people takes a long time: indeed, it goes on to the end of our lives.

To think that we know everything and nothing can change, is to die before our proper time, because living itself *is* growing and understanding. The friends in this book are beginning to grasp this. They are not content to end the quest for knowledge with a few lessons about sex and having babies. They are constantly turning over the ideas that come to them with each new experience of people in their lives.

If you have friends you enjoy talking to, you have something of great value. Friendship is the first step towards loving and being loved. It is a great gift that humans give to one another — indeed, this exchange of trust and confidence, this sharing of self with another is unique to human beings. It is worth your while to cultivate good friends and to learn how to be a good friend. It is an essential stage in the your own development.

Take a few years to work at this; do not rush into a relationship that has not passed through the months of discovery, testing, understanding and growth.

75

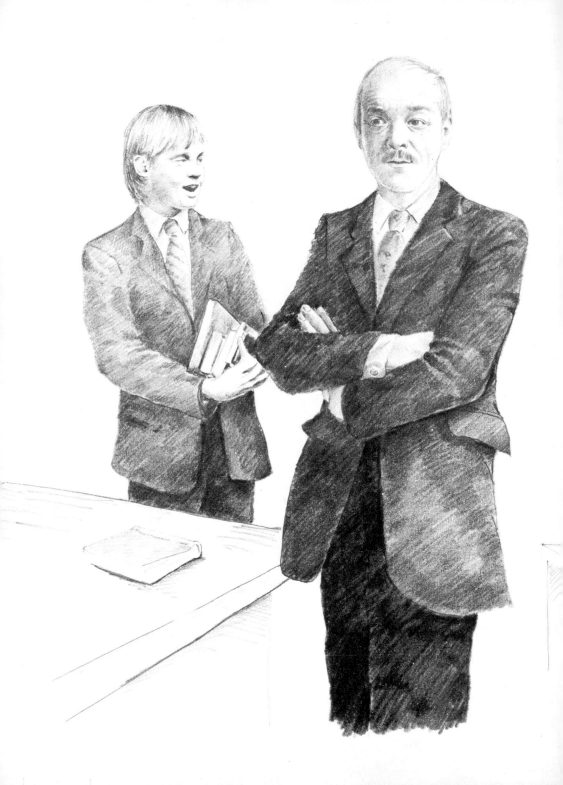

14

"Andy, you know you said to me, why don't I talk to Jenkins about things? Well, you were quite right. I was putting away books and things for him and we got talking. He's really good to talk to.

"I suppose it seemed easier to talk because we'd been to his house at Christmas. I asked him if he'd had a good time with all his family and then he asked me about my family. He didn't know I lived with my mum so I told him how I didn't know my dad, all I had ever had was my mum. He was really understanding. He said he always had a great admiration for one-parent families because they have to work so hard to be both parents at once to their children.

"He really seemed to know. I told him how I wished I had a father and how I envied all the friends I had who could talk to their fathers.

"He said I should think about how hard it had been for my mother, for she had to make all the decisions alone. When I was young she must often have been lonely and desperate and wished she could leave it all to someone else.

"Then he said the next best thing to a good father was to have some good friends and especially men like uncles or neighbours or someone I could talk to. Really he was saying that the person who matters most in your life is the person who cares about you and this could be anyone you know, not just your father."

"You're right, Nick. I know my father cares about me, but if he didn't I could go and talk to Chris—it's just having someone that's really important."

"You know Carl? Well, he's adopted. He told me once that he was

77

abandoned when he was a baby and then put in a home. Then his "adopted parents" came, visited him and eventually adopted him. He thinks the world of them."

"Well there you are, that's what I'm saying. Parents are not always the people who love you most. Whoever cares for you and brings you up—they're the people who matter to you."

"Parents are still the best people; after all, you are their child."

"Yes, but they have to want you and love you as well as just being parents. The way they go on at you sometimes it's hard to imagine they ever wanted you – never mind love you!"

"Jenkins says that's just because they do care about you. If you didn't matter to them, what would be the point of them telling you what to do or how to behave – they just wouldn't care what happened to you.

"He told me that when his eldest left home to share a flat with three other young people, she thought it was perfect freedom – no more rules or questions about who you are with or where you are going – she felt absolutely free to do just as she pleased.

"Then one night she stayed out at a party all night and her mates rang the police about four in the morning and said she was missing. When she got home they were all mad at her for not saying where she was or when she would be home. They'd had a whole lot of students in the area being attacked at night and they'd really got worried.

"Then she realised that it wasn't just parents being fussy – it was really caring about people, and it doesn't matter who you live with, you have a responsibility to tell them. If you don't want people to worry about you, you are really saying you don't want friends."

"Well I want friends, but I don't want them worrying about me."

"Would you worry about me if I got into trouble?"

"I'd want to help if I could."

"Well all I'm saying is other people – your friends – would want to help you if they could."

"You can't be a friend and not have a friend: it involves two people. You can't love nothing. You have to love someone and, straight away, that someone is involved with you."

"How did we get into this? All of a sudden everyone's getting serious."

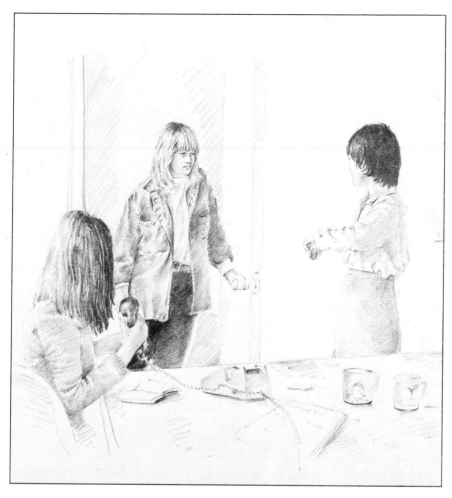

"It's a long time since we went down to the tree."

"Funny, I just thought the same—something to do with Andy saying how serious we are."

"That's what comes with growing up, you didn't have all these problems to work out before."

"It's all those films and talks you get in school — you're better off without adolescence!"

"Idiot! You can't choose not to grow up."

79

"Well anyway, the reason I started about old Jenkins is that when we'd talked about parents and things, he said perhaps we all had some things we'd like to talk about and would it be a good idea if he gave us some of his lesson time to ask a few questions and just talk about any worries we had – and I said, yes, I thought so, and I'd ask you."

And they all agreed that what was needed was time and freedom to discuss 'just anything'.

*   *   *

Talking to a trusted adult is very valuable in your youth. However good your relationship is with your parents, it is good to share some of your ideas with a teacher or a counsellor or a Youth Club leader. These people have all spent a great deal of time learning about young people and working with them. Sometimes a young person worries about things like masturbation or homosexuality, and if he or she asks their parents they too get worried, perhaps because they do not mix with enough young people to see that it is a normal and general anxiety among many of them.

Another advantage is that in a small group each person may raise a different question and the group learn from each other. You will also find that you are not alone—several people may be sharing your worries and that helps you. For instance, Nick discovered in the group discussion that .at least three other people were from broken families and they really shared their feelings about that. The rest of the group also learnt how to appreciate the difficulties of others and also how much they owed to their own families.

Here are some of the questions and discussions that were raised in the group, and how Jenkins dealt with them. Facts are facts, but questions about morality have to be thought out carefully. We have always to be careful not to let our feelings get in the way of clear thinking. These are two separate functions when dealing with the right and wrong of things. The *facts* which make a certain *behaviour* right or wrong have to be examined with our intelligence and reason. *Feelings* and sympathy are what we have for the *person* or persons involved.

For example, if somebody steals, our intelligence should tell us that this is very wrong behaviour, and our feelings should help us towards sympathy and understanding of the person. But we cannot confuse the two things and say stealing was good because the person was poor. You will see how this applies to some of the boys' questions.

How does a girl know when she's pregnant?

Usually, the first sign she has is when her periods stop. You remember the chapter about girls and how they change to women? In that you will see, if you turn back, that when the egg (ovum) is not fertilised it dies and the lining of blood tissue in the womb comes away. This happens fairly regularly each month. Now if the egg becomes fertilised – that is when a sperm from the father enters into it – the egg will bed itself down in the lining of the womb. A new life begins to grow inside the mother and she has no period for the nine months it takes for the baby to develop.

There are other signs as well, like the breasts getting firmer and rather tender, and sometimes some sickness early in the morning. But usually the first indication is the stopping of the periods.

What are these adverts about do your own pregnancy test?

That is a little kit you can buy at a chemist. It contains certain chemicals to which you add a sample of the woman's urine and the colour will show whether she is pregnant. Doctors and clinics use this method to confirm the fact if their patient says she thinks she is pregnant. But usually the woman wouldn't suspect this until after she has missed a period.

You keep saying the 'mother' and the 'father' as though they were married, but I know a young girl at school who has a baby.

However young she is, if she has a baby she is a mother and the boy responsible for making her pregnant is a father.

The fact that you think of a mother or father as being older, married people, shows that you have a good idea of the responsibilities that go with parenthood.

81

A mother and a father have to care, together, for any life they have created. They are responsible for giving the baby a home and a future with them. It is a very serious responsibility because the baby can have no control over this situation. He doesn't choose to be born and therefore a mother and father should consider together whether they want to take this on.

Sometimes young people have not thought about this at all. Perhaps they have never discussed it at home or in school as you are doing. They just think of 'sex' as something you do for pleasure: they do not think how closely it is tied to the creation of life, in fact, designed for this very purpose. The pleasure is the bonus you get for accepting responsibility for each other and the outcome of your sexual relationship—which could be a baby.

If young people have not worked this out, then they could find themselves having intercourse just as a part of 'necking' or 'petting'. These are words you use to describe kissing and cuddling and holding a girl very close to you. But if you do too much of this it gets out of your control. Young boys and girls get so involved in this kind of 'love-play' that they cannot stop the ultimate climax; then, 'accidentally', the girl may become pregnant.

Can you imagine being born unwanted, with two young parents who have no time for you, no plan for your future and probably no interest in each other?

Very often the boy has little or no interest in the girl, in the sense of a wife or mother. She was just a 'date', someone to go out with. He becomes frightened by the responsibility of what he has done and his inability to cope with it, so he leaves the girl to the care of her family and tries to forget all about it.

For the girl it is not so easy. She certainly can't forget about being pregnant. However kind her family is about taking care of her and the baby, there is still a great deal of hurt and unhappiness to be gone through.

Most parents look forward with pleasure to their children being married and presenting them with grandchildren. There is a proper time for these family celebrations. There is certainly no celebration about the arrival of a baby in a family in the unexpected fashion that we are talking about.

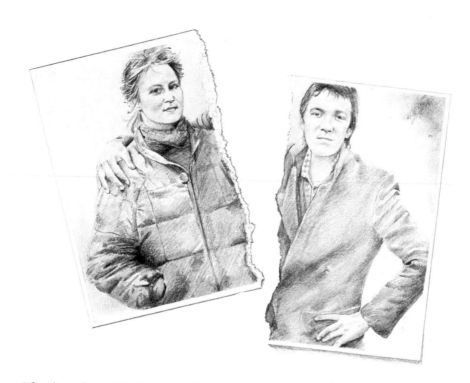

That's a bit old fashioned, people are much more broadminded about girls having babies nowadays.

This is one of these questions I mentioned in the beginning of this discussion, where you have to separate your feelings from the reasons. Most people still believe a baby should be born into a family with a home, where there is a mother and a father who both care about the child. They believe that the couple should be mature enough to accept full responsibility for this and to take on the role of parents.

Our society is built around this idea of family units and our laws are designed to help and protect and support it. When it breaks down we try to make laws to replace the care of the parents. When children are put 'in care', the home in which they live tries to imitate, as nearly as possible, normal family life. So we still uphold the principle of the family.

What has changed considerably is our attitude to the mother and baby. Society realises how innocent is the child in this situation.

People no longer look down on the child as though he or she were to blame. They try to love and care for the child and make up for the lack of parental love.

The girl, too, needs love and acceptance if she is to become a warm and loving mother to her baby. We have a responsibility as caring human beings to help one another. But you should not confuse this with the idea that it doesn't matter. However much we try to help the one-parent family there is always a sadness that it is in some way an incomplete family.

Why doesn't she get the baby adopted?

Quite often this does happen. But it is not an easy decision. Other people may see it as the simplest solution, but when you are the girl and you feel the life growing in you and then you give birth and the baby is laid in your arms, you may feel a great longing to keep this baby. Very few people give up their babies without pain and tears.

Why don't they have an abortion, then all this wouldn't happen?

Abortion means ending the life in the womb. Many people consider this is just as serious as killing a baby.

It is such a serious decision that people who think they want an abortion will discuss it with friends, doctors, priests, counsellors. They are often very confused and worried and looking for help. There are organisations run by people who are strongly opposed to abortion, who will help the mothers through their pregnancy and then help with adoption of the baby.

There are clinics where women or girls may go to have an abortion with medical supervision. There are different methods used for this, but all the methods have the same purpose, which is to kill the embryo or foetus in the womb and then to cause the womb to cast out the foetus and the womb lining.

If you turn back to the pages about the growth of the baby in the womb, you can see what stages are reached at each month and how quickly the organs and features take shape. If there is growth then there is certainly life.

People who agree with abortions usually say that it is a life-cell, but not a person. They believe it is only a person after birth when it can live apart from the mother. But if the parents are longing for a baby and really planned to have one, he becomes part of their lives from the time of conception. A baby in that case is very much a person to the parents right from the beginning of the pregnancy.

People who have abortions do not allow themselves to think of the baby in the womb as a person, for that would make it impossible for them to go through with the abortion. Even when they have made the decision it is not a happy time. Frequently there are after-effects which leave the woman sad and depressed. Sometimes it affects her desire to have children at a later date.

Wouldn't it be better not to get pregnant? I mean why can't they use a contraceptive?

That would certainly seem a more responsible way of dealing with their problem.

A contraceptive, in case some of you are wondering, is anything used to prevent the sperm from reaching the ovum and so fertilising the egg.

Sometimes the woman uses the contraceptive. The most commonly used one is the pill which I'm sure you have all read about at sometime. The pill contains hormones which prevent the ovaries from releasing the egg each month – just like the hormone which does this when a woman becomes pregnant. That is how the scientists learnt about this, by studying the effects of hormones on women at various times in their lives.

There are also sheaths which a man can wear. This is a very delicate rubber cover which slides over the penis and prevents the semen from going into the womb.

Then there are devices that a woman can fit in her vagina or womb.

All of these methods have their failures but they certainly lessen the likelihood of pregnancy.

A woman also has her own natural cycle by which she can regulate her sexual activity. There are times in the month between each period when she cannot conceive a baby and also a time at which it is very likely that she would conceive. She can work this out for herself with the help of a thermometer and by studying how her body behaves during each monthly cycle.

But with all these methods there is still the necessity to make responsible decisions, and not just 'leave it to chance'.

Which takes me back to your original question. Birth control would solve some people's problems, but not the casual boy/girl affair that I described where the youngsters only set out for a date and some necking. Nothing is farther from their minds than the possibility of having a baby and so of course nothing is planned or discussed about these matters.

So what can they do then if they don't want any trouble?

'They' could be 'you' at any time in the next few years. That is why I'm suggesting you think it out now before the situation arises.

If you make up your mind that going out with a girl is not going to include sexual intercourse then you are much less likely to get into that situation.

You can only make that kind of decision if you really have values—for instance, if you think the marriage relationship is a really special one that you want to experience with one special person, your wife.

Think of the girl—if she puts herself in your care for an evening she should be able to trust you. Her parents have allowed her to go out with you so they also trust you.

Then there is the value you set on yourself. Are you a man in full control of himself? Are you a boy who is not yet responsible? Are you ruled by your feelings and 'urges' or can you respond to a higher demand of self-control?

How do you get experience then?

Did you have any experience of life before you were born? Of course not. You learnt by living it a little at a time according to the age you were.

86

Sexual love is part of a life together. It is not your personal experience but a 'together' experience. So you learn about it by living a life together over many years. Love-making is a skill, an art, it grows better with each year you spend together. That is why most people still think marriage is the best school for learning about love.

When two people love each other they don't check out each other's experience, they don't even want to know who else has loved the person and what that was about. Each just wants reassurance that he or she is the person most loved by the other, and that is enough to begin their life together. So don't be taken in by all these magazine articles you read about your prowess as a lover and how to gain experience before making a decision to marry.

I can assure you that your wife will want you to experience her uniqueness for you. She has no wish to be graded somewhere in your record book A to E.

You keep talking about 'when you're married' but some people don't get married – they don't believe in all that church business.

Well I have already said a little about society and how it is organised in family units. In the same way it is easier for all kinds of legal reasons, documents, allowances, benefits and so on if couples get legally married.

You don't have to go to a church for this, you can marry in a Registry Office. You are, that way, making a public statement with witnesses, about your intention to live together and respect one another and be responsible for one another.

People who marry in church are making exactly the same kind of public statement, but they believe they will need help from God to keep their promises. So they ask for blessing and prayers from the priest or minister and those present. In a way it is a double statement. One thing is about what they want to do for each other and the other is an acknowledgement of God's involvement in their lives and their commitment to that.

Then there are people who say, 'It is quite enough that we promise one another and just stay together. That way we are absolutely free to stay or to go whichever pleases us.'

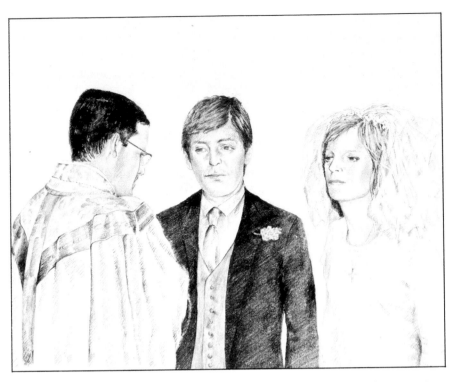

If they stay together for ever, and bring up a family, they are just as much married as any couple who go through a legal form of marriage. We are talking here about the relationship in marriage—the reality of the union, not its legal recognition.

But if the intention is to opt out whenever they choose, then it is not an honest relationship. When someone says, 'I love you' to another person, it implies 'for ever' – no one ever says, 'I'll love you for a week, or maybe for five years.' And so each partner in this 'free' situation lives in dread of the end. There is no security, and indeed no freedom, because you are afraid to be yourself, afraid that every little argument or difference will finish the agreement.

Getting married is only the beginning, a ceremony to start a new way of living. People have 'lived together' – man and woman – since time began. If you want to invent a new name for that there's nothing to stop you, but most people call it marriage.

What is a homosexual?

Everything you have read in this book has been about the love a man and woman have for each other, which usually leads to marriage and having children. That is the way most people are made, and the future of the human race depends upon this.

A homosexual is unable to experience this kind of sexual love for a person of the opposite sex. He or she may only have these feelings about people of his own sex. If we are talking about a woman we use the word 'lesbian'.

There is still a great deal to learn about the reasons why some people are homosexual; doctors and psychologists are always looking for greater understanding about this and for ways of helping this group of people to lead fully contented lives. For the present they have to live their own kind of life in the best way they can for personal fulfilment. They must accept themselves as they are.

We help them most by accepting each one as a person in his or her own right, likeable, lovable, and truly human. We must also be truly ourselves in relation to them. That means being natural, behaving as you would towards any friend or acquaintance. A homosexual person has as much right to courtesy and respect as a heterosexual (someone attracted to the opposite sex)—we are all groups in the human family.

The problem of homosexuality is often discussed in magazines and on television. Plays and stories are written to try and understand how it affects people's lives. Homosexuals form clubs and groups and say a great deal about themselves in public. All this makes it appear to be a 'fashion' scene.

Some young people get caught up in all this and begin to worry about themselves.

I've read about people who are homosexual and who get married and have a family.

Yes, some people have both kinds of sexuality in their nature. There's no clear line which divides those who are, from those who are not.

How do I know if I am a homosexual?

At your age it is very unlikely that you have completed the development of your 'maleness'. You are all still growing into men. During that period you often find the friends you like best are of your own sex. Sometimes they may be older than you—someone to admire or copy, or just someone you enjoy being with.

That is quite normal, it is a pity not to have such friendships just because you think people will say you are homosexual.

If you worry about things like that it will make you shy and unsociable. You have a lot of years to grow and develop and explore friendships and discover who you are. Most people are heterosexual and make normal happy marriages. At your present age you just need to be natural and honest about your friendships and do nothing that would make you lose your self-respect.

If strangers approach you in the street or in a public lavatory, making suggestions you do not like, just walk away and do not become involved with them. That is just common sense, since you don't know them. If they persist in following you tell them you will tell the police if they do not leave you alone. And make sure you do tell the police or at least your parents so that they can decide what to do. It is better to tell this kind of incident to someone else, like a parent or teacher, because it is the kind of secret that can grow into a big worry if you don't get rid of it by talking.

Why are some children born handicapped?

Well that could be a fault in the genes. You read about those in your biology lessons. You remember there is a gene for absolutely every part of you – hair, skin, limbs, etc. Of course accidents causing brain damage or physical disability can make a healthy person handicapped at any time of his or her life.

So it isn't smoking or drinking that causes it?

Of course not. There are some handicaps you can do nothing about: even the doctors do not yet understand the cause. But smoking and drinking causes damage in another way.

You remember how the baby in the womb is attached to the placenta by the umbilical cord, a kind of life line for blood and oxygen and food? Now obviously if the mother smokes or drinks,

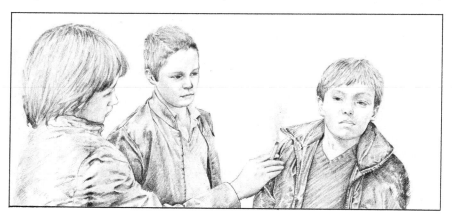

nicotine or alcohol will enter the blood stream and pass through the cord to the baby. Lots of expectant mums have an occasional drink for a special celebration or perhaps an occasional cigarette. The blood stream can cope with that but it cannot cope with an excess of it and then the baby's future health may be harmed.

What's the difference between rape and seduction?

To put it simply, seduction is tempting a young girl to have sexual intercourse with you when she is not old enough or mature enough to understand how serious this is. The law is designed to protect girls from this, by stating an age below which any boy or man who has intercourse with her can be charged with a criminal offence. It is no excuse in law to say that you didn't know.

Rape is forcing a girl or woman, of any age, to have intercourse against her wish. It is a much more violent crime and does a great deal of damage to the victim physically and psychologically. Society often makes excuses for young people in a case of seduction, but never for rape—it is something which every normal human being feels very strongly about. It is considered a crime against the dignity of man and woman, and a man must be a pretty sick kind of person to do it.

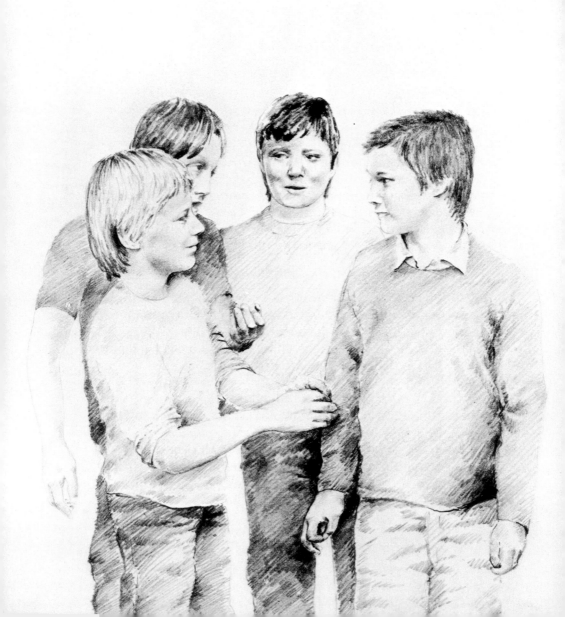

Conclusion

All that discussion gave the boys plenty to think about. Andy, Nick, Pete and Tony have learnt a lot about themselves in this last year. They have also learnt quite a lot about other people.

Their opinions about some people have changed and they begin to understand what adult standards and values are all about. They will still question everything and work it out for themselves. The difference is that less anger flies around now and more discussion takes place.

Everything is not as simple for them as it was a few years back. They have to accept more responsibility for what they do. They have to consider how they affect other people rather than just what pleases them.

The harder they work at this the greater becomes the relationship with their families and friends. They begin to feel the pleasure of being trusted by parents and taken into consideration like adults. Soon even the law will consider them legally responsible for their action even though they are still in their 'teens'.

All this may be just where you are now. If you feel that you have 'grown up' with the boys and taken on some of these responsibilities then you are well on the way to making a man of yourself—and your family happy and proud of you.

The greatest gift you can give to your parents is this proof that all their caring for you has been worthwhile.

Perhaps you are much younger than the boys in the book and are only beginning to wonder about all these things. If that is so, keep this book where you can use it. Go back to it whenever you want to check out information or find an answer. Talk about what is in the book with your parents or with a teacher, or even with your friends.

Some parts of the book will be more interesting than others depending on your age. As you grow up, the message of love and human understanding will seem more important than the actual facts and information. Read it again before you leave school and check out how you have changed since you first received the book. You may be surprised to find that little bits about girls and behaviour will stand out this time when they meant nothing to you a few years back.

Whatever age you are, one thing is certain – you will get older. So enjoy growing up: let it happen in its own time. Do not rush into manhood without noticing your youth. Each stage of your life is interesting, but the years of your adolescence are filled with hopes and dreams and expectations, such as you will never experience again.